# Enduring Legacy

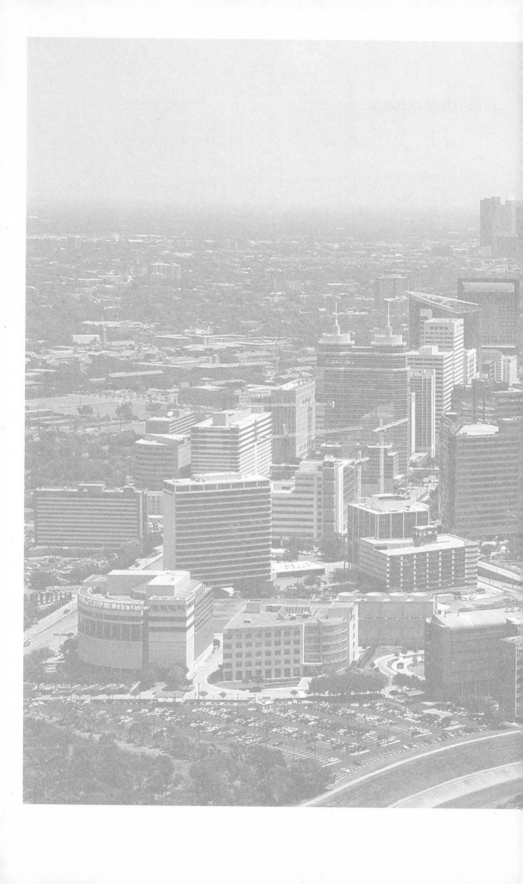

# Enduring Legacy

## The M. D. Anderson Foundation & the Texas Medical Center

WILLIAM HENRY KELLAR

*Foreword by George H. W. Bush & James A. Baker, III*

TEXAS A&M UNIVERSITY PRESS | *College Station*

Manufactured in the United States of America
This paper meets the requirements
of ANSI/NISO Z39.48-1992
(Permanence of Paper).
Binding materials have been chosen for durability.

LIBRARY OF CONGRESS CATALOGING-IN-PUBLICATION DATA

Kellar, William Henry, 1952– author.

   Enduring legacy : The M. D. Anderson Foundation and the Texas Medical Center
/ William Henry Kellar ; foreword by George H. W. Bush and James A. Baker, III. —
First edition.
       pages cm
   Includes bibliographical references and index.
   ISBN 978-1-62349-131-4 (cloth : alk. paper) —
   ISBN 978-1-62349-140-6 (e-book)
   1. Texas Medical Center—History. 2. M. D. Anderson Foundation
(Houston, Tex.)—History. 3. Anderson, Monroe D. (Monroe Dunaway),
1873–1939. 4. Medical centers—Texas—Houston—History.
5. Houston (Tex.)—History. I. Title.
   RA982.H62 T49
   362.1109764'1411—dc23
   2013035948

*To Monroe Dunaway Anderson*
*and to all the others who helped build the Texas Medical Center*

# Contents

List of Illustrations    ix

Foreword, by George H. W. Bush and James A. Baker, III    xi

Preface    xv

Introduction    xxi

Chapter 1. Early Houston: A Magnet for Entrepreneurs in
Business and Medicine    1

Chapter 2. Building the Fortune: Anderson, Clayton & Company    24

Chapter 3. The Legal Team: Fulbright, Crooker, Freeman & Bates    48

Chapter 4. Legacy: Creating the M. D. Anderson Foundation    66

Chapter 5. Bold Vision: First Steps toward Building a Medical
Center    83

Chapter 6. Building Blocks: Baylor University College of Medicine    98

Chapter 7. "One of the Greatest Medical Centers Ever Developed"    117

Chapter 8. A Building Boom in the Texas Medical Center    137

Chapter 9. The Biggest Medical Center in the World    161

Epilogue: The Enduring Legacy of Monroe Dunaway Anderson    187

Appendix 1. M. D. Anderson Foundation Trustees, 1936–2013    201

Appendix 2. Texas Medical Center Member Institutions    203

Notes    207

A Note on Sources    233

Index    237

# Illustrations

Houston, ca. 1868   8

Baptist Sanitarium, ca. 1908   17

Hermann Hospital, ca. 1926   19

Frank E. Anderson   28

William L. Clayton   32

Benjamin Clayton   33

Old Cotton Exchange Building   39

Monroe D. Anderson standing on cotton bales   42

R. C. Fulbright, ca. 1919   50

John H. Freeman   52

John H. Crooker in his World War I uniform   57

William B. Bates in his World War I uniform   59

Monroe D. Anderson in his later years   71

Horace M. Wilkins   76

Main house at The Oaks   85

Dr. Ernst W. Bertner as a young man   91

Julia Williams Bertner in her youth   92

Dr. Frederick C. Elliott   95

Dr. Walter H. Moursund   101

Sears, Roebuck warehouse on Buffalo Drive   114

Leland Anderson presenting the land deed to E. W. Bertner, 1946   124

Converted barracks at M. D. Anderson Hospital, 1947   128

Cullen Building, Baylor University College of Medicine, ca. 1946   130

Dr. E. W. Bertner receiving an honorary LLD degree, 1950   134

Construction at the Texas Medical Center, 1950   138

Texas Medical Center, aerial view, 1953   147

Leon Jaworski as a youth   155

Ben Taub Hospital, ca. 1963   158

Richard E. Wainerdi, president of the Texas Medical Center   163

University of Texas Medical School at Houston under construction, 1975   172

Texas Medical Center, 2011   184

Frederick C. Elliott, R. Lee Clark, and William B. Bates, 1970   193

John H. Freeman, 1978   195

# Foreword

There are many reasons why the two of us believe that Houston is a world-class city. Atop that list, of course, are the intelligent, innovative, and, above all, visionary people who have persevered to turn their city from a mudhole along Buffalo Bayou into a thriving metropolis that nurtures some of the finest institutions in the world. The vast expanses of outer space have been explored from Houston at the Johnson Space Center. The depths of the earth have been mined for energy by international leaders in that field with headquarters here. Great minds have been produced at Rice University and our city's other institutions of higher education. The list goes on and on. From construction of the Houston Ship Channel to building the world's first domed stadium, Houston has always strived to stay ahead of the curve—and it typically succeeds.

At the top of Houston's many accomplishments is the simple truth that much of the world's finest medical research and health care has been provided in this city. That began when the M. D. Anderson Foundation established the Texas Medical Center more than seventy years ago. As we in Texas like to say: "That's no brag, just fact." Today Houston is home to the biggest and one of the best medical centers ever known to mankind.

From research at the University of Texas M. D. Anderson Cancer Center to pediatric care at Texas Children's Hospital to innovative cardiac research at the Texas Heart Institute, no other medical center can boast of as many accomplishments. Add to this fourteen other hospitals, three medical schools, four nursing schools, and schools of dentistry, public health, and pharmacy, and you can quickly understand why the Texas Medical Center is recognized around the world for its quality patient care, teaching, research, and prevention of illness and injury.

The two of us are proud to write the foreword for this book, *Enduring Legacy: The M. D. Anderson Foundation and the Texas Medical Center*. William Henry Kellar's well-researched account of this unlikely success story chronicles step by step the medical center's steady march from vision to greatness. The author carefully weaves the medical center's growth with the history of this wonderful city in a thoughtful fashion that helps explain the symbiotic relationship between the two. It is a book worthy both of Houston and the Texas Medical Center.

This story begins with the vision of one man, banker and cotton trader Monroe Dunaway Anderson, who in 1936 established a charitable foundation for the purpose of providing better health care and to support other causes in Houston. Upon his death in 1939, he had bequeathed more than $19 million to the new M. D. Anderson Foundation. Its first gift was $1,000 to the Junior League Eye Fund for eyeglasses.

Soon enough, however, foundation trustees set upon their goal of building a "city of health." Led by attorneys William B. Bates and John H. Freeman and banker Horace M. Wilkins, Houston's civic leaders were sold on the idea of achieving the goal of transforming 134 acres around Hermann Hospital into a medical center. In 1941 they convinced the Texas Legislature to provide the funds to fulfill the dream of Bates, Freeman, and Houston physician Ernst W. Bertner to start the cancer research center that would be named after Anderson. The foundation matched the state's grant with land and money.

From this start grew the Texas Medical Center. Two years later, the foundation invited Baylor College of Medicine to move from Dallas to join the University of Texas Dental School as two important teaching institutions at the fledgling Texas Medical Center. What followed was simply fantastic as the center continued to grow and improve under the foundation's watchful eye and leadership.

Since then, the Texas Medical Center has been home base for legendary heart surgeons Michael DeBakey and Denton Cooley, who advanced cardiac medicine like no others before or since. Emil Freireich, who helped pioneer the first combination chemotherapy for cancer and successfully applied it to acute lymphoblastic leukemia in children, practiced at the Texas Medical Center. So did Katherine H. K. Hsu, who has made tremendous contributions to the treatment and prevention of tuberculosis. The same can be said for countless other medical experts who have been at the very top of their fields.

Accomplishments at the Texas Medical Center during the past

seven decades have been remarkable. So has the outstanding generosity provided by so many dedicated supporters. Time and time again, Houstonians have dug deep into their own pockets to make contributions that have made possible our medical center's growth. The result? Others have tried to duplicate what Houston has accomplished. None have succeeded.

The two of us are old enough to have seen the development of the Texas Medical Center from the dream of a local businessman and his lawyers to the impressive reality that it is today. And we can't help agreeing with a comment made by one Houston historian: "If the founders of the Texas Medical Center were here today, they'd look out across the vast expanse of hospitals and medical schools and streets that make up the medical center and say: 'I see it out there but I don't believe it.'"

Fortunately, the Texas Medical Center is out there. Bold and grand, it is a testament to the great city that is Houston.

George H. W. Bush and James A. Baker, III

# *Preface*

*Enduring Legacy: The M. D. Anderson Foundation and the Texas Medical Center,* a history of the M. D. Anderson Foundation, is a project with which I have been engaged in some manner for slightly more than ten years. Originally it began as a biography of Monroe Dunaway Anderson. But as time passed, the project evolved into a broader history of the cotton firm he cofounded, Anderson, Clayton & Company, with a view toward including a chapter on the Anderson Foundation as part of the firm's legacy. Over the years, I continued my research for this project as time permitted, taking advantage of opportunities to conduct interviews with key people or their close acquaintances and keeping a vigilant eye out for materials related to Anderson, Clayton as I researched other projects. During this time, apart from teaching and other work at the University of Houston, most of my research and writing centered on the history of the Texas Medical Center. As I became more familiar with the development of the medical center, I also began to acquire a better appreciation for the understated but crucial role that the M. D. Anderson Foundation played as the driving force behind the efforts to create and nurture this amazing complex and its member institutions.

Coincidentally, during the fall of 2007, my friend and colleague at the University of Houston's Center for Public History, Joseph A. Pratt, conducted an interview with Gibson Gayle Jr., who was at the time president of the M. D. Anderson Foundation. Pratt was interviewing notable Houstonians as part of both the university's Houston History Project and Mayor Bill White's Oral History of Houston. Following this interview, Gayle mentioned that the foundation was interested in having a history written that would focus primarily on the founding of the Texas Medical Center and the role the Anderson Foundation had in it. Knowing that I had been doing related research and also had written extensively about the medical center, Pratt contacted me about the project. Over the next few months he met several times with the trustees and reached an agreement by which the M. D. Anderson Foundation would provide a grant to the University of Houston's Center for Public History to fund the research, writing, and editing of a history of the Texas Medical Center and the foundation. Pratt and I collaborated on an outline for the proposed project, and I was selected to take the lead as it got under way.

In addition to conducting new research specifically for this project, I was able to draw upon my previous work, which included a series of related oral history interviews, and voluminous notes, transcripts, and photocopies that I had collected over the years. A significant portion of this information came from the private collection of W. Merrill Glasgow, for many years vice president of corporate planning and business development of Anderson, Clayton & Company. Glasgow had saved many documents related to the firm after it was sold, including copies of annual reports dating back to 1905, the year after the firm was established in Oklahoma City, and other original documents. He generously made his collection available to me and has since donated these documents to Special Collections at the University of Houston M. D. Anderson Library. Glasgow also introduced me to several surviving former executives of the company who graciously agreed to let me conduct oral history interviews with them. In addition to these materials, the Texas Medical Center had engaged historian Louis Marchiafava to interview several members of the board of directors, which added yet another resource from which I could draw. As I continued my work, archivist Philip Montgomery and historical collections assistant Alethea Drexler of the John P. McGovern Historical Collections and Research Center at the Texas Medical Center Library discovered the videotaped interviews conducted by N. Don Macon during the early 1970s. These interviews included sessions with many of the founders and early supporters of the Texas Medical Center. The McGovern Center permitted me to have the tapes converted to DVDs for viewing on modern equipment. Other research included both primary and secondary resources found in the collections of the Houston Metropolitan Research Center of the Houston Public Library, the John P. McGovern Historical Collections and Research Center of the Texas Medical Center Library, Special Collections of the University of Houston M. D. Anderson Library, the files of the M. D. Anderson Foundation, and various institutional websites on the Internet.

The final manuscript comprises ten chapters, including an epilogue, with a primary focus on events leading up to and including the founding era of the Texas Medical Center, from 1941 to 1962. It also includes a number of biographical sketches of key people who were well known to their contemporaries but whose contributions are increasingly lost to history apart from their names on buildings and streets in the city. The book begins with a brief overview of the development of Houston as a magnet for entrepreneurs and the evolution of public health in the city. Succeeding chapters focus on the rise of Anderson, Clayton & Company as a major global cotton firm, which in turn produced the fortune on which the M. D. Anderson Foundation was established; the role of the firm's attorneys at Fulbright, Crooker, Freeman & Bates in creating the M. D. Anderson Foundation; and the subsequent founding and development of the Texas Medical Center. A sixth chapter chronicles the issues and significance related to relocating the Baylor University College of Medicine from Dallas (1943) to become part of the Texas Medical Center in Houston. Chapter 7 examines the role of the Anderson Foundation and the medical center's first president, Dr. Ernst W. Bertner, during the organizational years until Bertner's premature death in 1950. Chapter 8 looks at his successor, Dr. Frederick C. Elliott, who worked closely with the foundation as the medical center experienced its first period of rapid growth and astonishing success. Chapter 9 provides a brief update on the Texas Medical Center since the founding era, and an epilogue provides an update on the M. D. Anderson Foundation and the many types of institutions it has supported through the years.

This study is based upon a variety of primary and secondary sources, some that have been used elsewhere and some that have never been accessed before this project. *Enduring Legacy*, then, provides a unique perspective on what has proved to be the indispensable role of the M. D. Anderson Foundation in the creation of the Texas Medical Center. It also provides a case study of how public and private institutions worked together to create a veritable city of health that became the largest medical complex in human history. This work fills a gap in the existing literature on Houston philanthropy and the creation of the Texas Medical Center. It will be useful to anyone who has an interest in the history of Houston, the Texas Medical Center, and the M. D. Anderson Foundation, or who is seeking biographical information on some of the civic leaders of the period. It also serves as a reminder that during these times of intense debate about the future of health care in the United States, the health care professionals of the Texas Medical Center stand largely untapped as a resource in the conversation.

This project would not have been possible without the support of the M. D. Anderson Foundation and the University of Houston's Center for Public History. I am especially grateful to the trustees of the Anderson Foundation and particularly to Gibson Gayle Jr. and Charles W. Hall for graciously making themselves available to be interviewed and for their help in locating files and other materials that proved essential in writing this history. My sincere thanks also go to Dr. Martin V. Melosi, executive director of the Center for Public History and Dr. Joseph A. Pratt, director of the Houston History Project, for their support of this endeavor. Over the years that I was doing my research for this project, Thomas Dunaway Anderson graciously provided access to his files of personal correspondence between his father, Frank E. Anderson, and his uncle, Monroe D. Anderson. He also furnished documents and other papers from his collection, including biographical articles he had researched and written about his famous "Uncle Mon." Thomas Anderson was a consummate gentleman, generous in sharing his time and very encouraging as I continued my work on this project. I am also deeply grateful to Dr. Mavis P. Kelsey Sr. for his encouragement and support for this project. Kelsey shared his recollections of key people and events in the development of the Texas Medical Center during formal interviews and in our many conversations over the years. His endorsement of my work helped open many doors as I continued my research for this project and other studies related to Houston's medical history. Also, special thanks to W. Merrill Glasgow for making available to me his private collection of Anderson, Clayton & Company materials.

There are many others who made substantial contributions to this project, including the people who participated in the oral history interviews. Dr. Richard E. Wainerdi, president and CEO of the Texas Medical Center, made time for me in his busy schedule on several occasions and was very supportive throughout the project. David M. Underwood, chairman of the Texas Medical Center's board of directors, Gibson Gayle Jr., past president of the M. D. Anderson Foundation, Charles W. Hall, the foundation's current president, and Mary Bates Bentsen, daughter of Col. William B. Bates, one of the original trustees of the foundation, were among those who agreed to be interviewed. Although not all interviewees were quoted in the text, their comments provided useful information and were very important in helping me to understand the context in which this history transpired. Their names and the dates of their interviews appear in the note on sources. Also indispensable to this project were Wanda Van Hook and Suzanne Mascola, who ably transcribed most of the oral history interviews, and historian Kimberly Youngblood, who helped in numerous ways as lead researcher and who also wrote some initial rough drafts of the introductory chapters. My colleague from several earlier projects, Elisabeth O'Kane Lipartito, brought her historical expertise and keen editorial skills to improve the manuscript. In addition, Elisabeth's cheerful demeanor and positive outlook were a source of great encouragement along the way. Leslie Richards proved to be invaluable as a researcher during the final phase of this project, tracking down obscure sources and finding answers to those pesky follow-up questions that often arise. Elizabeth Borst White, Pam Cornell, and, later, Philip Montgomery and Alethea Drexler of the McGovern Center guided me to key information and rare photographs in the medical center's vast collections. Administrative assistance for the project came from the very capable and unfailingly pleasant Kristin Deville, program coordinator at the Center for Public History. Finally, to the many others without whose help this project could not have been accomplished, my sincere and deepest thanks.

# Introduction

Located in Houston, the Texas Medical Center is the largest medical center in the world. Although the idea of building a medical complex in the Bayou City had been suggested occasionally during the 1920s and 1930s, it was the M. D. Anderson Foundation, established by Monroe Dunaway Anderson in 1936, that ultimately became the driving force behind creating and shaping the center of today. Indeed, this spectacular concentration of institutions dedicated to healing, medical research, and education took years to develop, and it arose in a rather unlikely setting on the Texas coastal plains, fifty miles inland from the Gulf of Mexico, on a tract of soggy land just south of downtown Houston. In considering this history of the M. D. Anderson Foundation, the Texas Medical Center, and the people who were the major players, one cannot help but ask: "Why Houston?" What first attracted the early settlers in the beginning? How is it that the little log cabin settlement on Buffalo Bayou grew to become such a thriving economic region that would both sow the seeds for and support a world-renowned medical center? Houston as a magnet for entrepreneurs is, in fact, part of the sequence of events that led first to the creation of the M. D. Anderson Foundation and later to the founding of the Texas Medical Center. This study will examine the confluence of events that led to creating these venerable institutions, the key people who played significant roles, and the historical setting in which both the foundation and the medical center have continued to thrive.

During the first century of its existence, Houston was not an easy place in which to live. It proved to be an environment rich in natural resources, however, strategically located to become a center of trade and conducive to the kind of business success that encouraged firms both large and small to locate here. From the city's inception in 1836, Houston has been a business-friendly community that attracted men and women who saw opportunity and who brought with them both an entrepreneurial spirit and the bold thinking that enabled them to dream large. Not all of them succeeded in their business endeavors, but many did, and most of these people possessed both self-interest and a sense of civic virtue that inspired them to give back to the community that had nurtured their success. City leaders emerged in other burgeoning professions in the Bayou City: physicians, who were instrumental in improving the city's public health care; lawyers, who played an integral part in helping the city's growing business community develop on a sound footing; and bankers, who found creative ways to finance both public and private endeavors. So, as Houston began to develop, cotton traders and men in the timber and transportation industries helped the city grow economically, which in turn attracted others who continued to move the city forward. Later it was pioneers in the oil industry, petrochemicals, space technology, and researchers in science and medicine, all bringing their dreams, ideas, and energy.

Many of the men and women in the business and professional community exercised great influence over the direction of Houston as the city grew in size and population and as it matured in its institutions and amenities. Physicians, lawyers, bankers, and business professionals of every type served in leadership capacities as mayors, city council members, county officials, and leaders in their professional associations. Several of the names that appear in this study are representative of these men and women who believed strongly in building a better Houston both for themselves and for succeeding generations. They volunteered their time and in many cases donated much of the wealth they had earned through their business endeavors, all with the ultimate goal of making Houston into a world-class city. Individually, their stories are intriguing and adventurous, but collectively, they developed a "can-do" community spirit that encouraged the innovation, creativity, cooperation, and plain old hard work ethic that led to their own success and to the development of Houston as a burgeoning, cosmopolitan, international city.

Early on, these civic leaders envisioned a great city, and they found ways to inspire their fellow Houstonians to join them in supporting their grand ideas and worthy causes, often with amazing results. By creating their own innovative mechanisms for matching private and public funding, they frequently achieved the impossible, from digging the Houston Ship Channel and creating a deepwater seaport—fifty miles from the sea—to later building the first air-conditioned, domed sports stadium. And it was into this entrepreneurial milieu that Monroe Dunaway Anderson first arrived in 1907: the place where his firm, Anderson, Clayton & Company, achieved its great success and where he decided to bequeath the wealth he had accumulated in his adopted hometown when he formed the philanthropic foundation that bears his name. Monroe Anderson, in launching his foundation, also established an entity that in time would bring together some of Houston's most talented, civic-minded leaders from the legal, medical, banking, construction, and business communities in an ambitious quest to build a "city of health" that would be second to none. After his death in 1939, it was the trustees of the M. D. Anderson Foundation—two lawyers, William B. Bates and John H. Freeman, and a banker, Horace M. Wilkins—who pulled together this coalition of Houston's civic leaders and inspired their support in Houston's most noble endeavor, creating the Texas Medical Center.[1]

To understand the historical context in which both the M. D. Anderson Foundation and the Texas Medical Center were established, chapter 1 examines the notion of Houston as a magnet for entrepreneurs and the role of the city's physicians, who provided for the community's health and frequently took on the responsibilities of community leadership. As Houston continued to grow, it attracted more businesses, including the cotton firm of Anderson, Clayton & Company. Chapter 2 focuses on the men who established the firm and its ensuing success that made all of them, including Monroe Anderson, very wealthy. As Houston's businesses expanded, they required the assistance of good lawyers, who helped create sound organizational structures and also connected local companies to the larger national business scene. Anderson, Clayton & Company was no different and became one of the first clients of Clarence Fulbright's Houston law firm (known today as Fulbright & Jaworski LLP), which in 1919 became Fulbright & Crooker; in 1924, Fulbright, Crooker & Freeman; and in 1940, Fulbright, Crooker, Freeman & Bates, the name by which it was known during most of the period covered in this history. The firm's attorneys also played a key role as community leaders and later as trustees of the M. D. Anderson Foundation and founders of the Texas Medical Center. Chapter 3 explores the background of the lawyers who created the firm, particularly the attorneys who, with Monroe Anderson, formed the first board of trustees for the M. D. Anderson Foundation. Chapter 4 completes the historical background by looking at the creation of the foundation in 1936 and Anderson's death three years later. While his will went through probate and a review by the Internal Revenue Service, a series of events began in Texas that ultimately coincided with the foundation's quest for a project that would fulfill its mission and secure Monroe Anderson's legacy.

In 1941 the Texas Legislature authorized the creation of a state cancer hospital under the auspices of the University of Texas. This in turn served as the catalyst to a series of events, steps that led ultimately to locating the new hospital in Houston, naming it to honor M. D. Anderson, and making it the cornerstone of what would become his foundation's signature achievement, the Texas Medical Center. Chapter 5, then, looks at the step-by-step development of the medical center from its inception through the stages of its initial development, including the central role of the Anderson Foundation's board of trustees. As local medical institutions began to show interest in the new center, the Anderson trustees and their medical advisor, Dr. Ernst W. Bertner, worried that they needed a medical school to join the coalition of the cancer hospital and the new University of Texas dental school. When it appeared that the Baylor University College of Medicine in Dallas might be forced to close, decisive action by the Anderson Foundation's trustees saved the medical school and brought it to Houston to become a key component of their future medical center. Chapter 6, therefore, examines the events that led to the medical school's relocation, first to temporary facilities in an old Sears warehouse and later into the first new building constructed in the Texas Medical Center.

As World War II came to a close in 1945, the wartime moratorium on new construction ended, and planning for the Texas Medical Center began in earnest. When the Anderson Foundation took the unusual step of forming a separate entity to manage the new medical complex, the obvious choice to become the first president of Texas Medical Center, Inc. (TMC), was the charismatic local physician who had been involved with its planning almost from the beginning, E. W. Bertner. Chapter 7 follows Bertner as he began laying the groundwork for a dynamic, lasting medical center, his heroic personal fight to survive cancer, and his untimely death from the dread disease in 1950. Following Bertner's death, the Anderson Foundation continued its support of the medical center and its growing list of member institutions. While the TMC board of directors engaged in a search for Bertner's successor, Dr. Frederick C. Elliott, dean of the UT dental school and one of the first to sign the charter that established the Texas Medical Center, assumed the role as interim leader. By 1952, the directors recognized that he was the logical successor to Bertner and formally appointed Elliott as executive director. During Elliott's decadelong tenure, the Texas Medical Center experienced its first building boom and began its rise to national prominence. Chapter 8 provides a look at Elliott's leadership, the spectacular growth of the medical center, and the M. D. Anderson Foundation's continuing role in supporting this enterprise. Elliott's retirement in 1962 also marked the end of what could be described as the "founding era" of the Texas Medical Center. During the fifty years since, the Texas Medical Center has expanded in size and in the number of member institutions—from 134 acres to more than 1,300 and from a handful of members to more than fifty. Chapter 9 provides an overview of the changes, growth, and amazing success that have made the Texas Medical Center the largest medical complex in the world.

The M. D. Anderson Foundation has continued its unfailing support of the Texas Medical Center throughout its history. In addition to financial support through philanthropic grants, the foundation's trustees have served regularly on the TMC board and as directors of other member institutions. Although the Texas Medical Center is the foundation's most spectacular achievement, it is hardly the only beneficiary of the foundation's work. Thus, the final chapter, an epilogue, provides a general overview of the foundation's work and the various types of institutions it has supported during its seventy-plus-year history. Over the years, the trustees have been prudent in their role as stewards of Monroe Anderson's original bequest, some $19 million, and have skillfully managed the assets so that the foundation has been able to give some $270 million in grants to hundreds of worthy organizations, including the member institutions of the Texas Medical Center.

This introduction would be remiss if it did not address two areas of confusion related to the Texas Medical Center and to the M. D. Anderson Foundation. Although most Houstonians are familiar with the

Texas Medical Center, occasionally there is some confusion about exactly how to define this institution and to understand how it functions. David M. Underwood, chairman of the Texas Medical Center's board of directors, observed that people generally mean one of three things when they talk about it. "It could mean the geographic location," stated Underwood. "Everybody thinks of the Texas Medical Center as our main campus." He refers here to the complex that began on the original 134 acres south of downtown Houston. Underwood also noted that people sometimes think of the group—over fifty member institutions—while others envision the corporation, Texas Medical Center. In fact, all of these ideas define the Texas Medical Center as it exists today. It encompasses some 1,300 acres of land, which now includes a Mid-Campus and a South Campus. There are over fifty independent member institutions that, as Dr. Richard E. Wainerdi, president and CEO of the Texas Medical Center, stated, "have come together and decided that there is an advantage to combining competition and collaboration in a productive way." As discussed in chapter 9, some of these institutions also have global outreach programs. In addition to the member institutions, there is the corporate entity, Texas Medical Center, Inc. (TMC), now known simply as Texas Medical Center. As planning for the Texas Medical Center evolved during World War II, the M. D. Anderson Foundation trustees also organized an independent corporation, Texas Medical Center, Inc., to manage the land, apportion tracts to individual member institutions, and enforce the covenants that would ensure this city of health would remain exactly that, a nonprofit center in which nonprofit, health-related institutions could work to conduct research, train health care professionals, and provide improved care to patients. This corporate entity, Texas Medical Center, also promotes communication, collaboration, and cooperation between member institutions. All of this means that not only has the Texas Medical Center grown to become the largest medical complex in the world, but it also is unique in that there is not one singular administrative structure or university system that governs all of its institutions.[2]

Occasionally, a similar confusion arises about the M. D. Anderson Foundation and the University of Texas M. D. Anderson Cancer Center. It is important to note that they are two separate, distinct institutions. At no time has the foundation ever exercised any administrative control over the cancer hospital or its operations. As discussed in chapter 4, the Anderson Foundation provided an initial grant to match the state appropriation when the cancer hospital was first established in 1941, offered a temporary home, and later made available a tract of land for a permanent site if the University of Texas board of regents agreed to name the hospital after Monroe D. Anderson and locate it in Houston. The regents agreed, and the M. D. Anderson Hospital for Cancer Research, as it was first known, became the inspiration and cornerstone for a medical center to be built in Houston.

This book, then, primarily is a chronicle of the events and the key people that led first to creating the M. D. Anderson Foundation and of its central role in later founding the Texas Medical Center. How and why all of this happened to take place in Houston is an integral piece of the story. In the end, the generous gift of a rather shy yet talented Houston businessman created the M. D. Anderson Foundation. But it was the men Anderson first chose as trustees of his foundation and their successors who, in remaining faithful to his charge, exercised bold vision and dynamic leadership to create one of the most magnificent places of healing and good works in human history. Today the Texas Medical Center is many things, but it also stands as a tribute to the integrity of his foundation's trustees and as a symbol of the enduring legacy of Monroe D. Anderson.

# Enduring Legacy

# Chapter 1

## Early Houston

### A Magnet for Entrepreneurs in Business and Medicine

*"The pioneer physicians of Houston, long on the art of medicine and short on the science, not only battled disease but other vicissitudes of the times."*

—Walter H. Moursund, MD, Dean,
Baylor University College of Medicine, 1923–1953

Houston, Texas, was founded in August 1836 by two land speculators, brothers Augustus C. and John Kirby Allen. From the beginning, the city has attracted ambitious people, many of whom built successful businesses and accumulated great wealth. Along with a driving ambition, the Allen brothers also possessed a civic mindedness that inspired them to give back to the community and leave the city a better place for those who followed in their footsteps. This spirit of hard work, civic obligation, and generous giving can be found first in the men responsible for establishing the M. D. Anderson Foundation and later in those who led the way in creating what ultimately became the largest medical complex in the world, the Texas Medical Center. The very founding of Houston typified the spirit of entrepreneurship that would come to be associated with the city in later decades. Contrary to early advertising, however, Houston was hardly a garden spot and, with its location fifty miles inland from the Gulf of Mexico, not a place that seemed destined to be a major port of trade. It is reasonable, then, to ask what attracted so many hardworking, visionary people to Houston, and how did the largest medical center in the world come to be established here, in what one might have considered the most unlikely of places? The story of the M. D. Anderson Foundation and the development of the Texas Medical Center are unique in American history. In order to understand fully the significance of how the Texas Medical Center would be created and fostered in such a wild yet wonderful place, it is important to look briefly at the economic origins of the city, the growing concern for public health in the community, and the leadership role that the city's physicians and businessmen have taken during the course of Houston's history.

Houston's founders, the Allen brothers, demonstrated savvy marketing ability when they named their new town to honor Gen. Sam Houston, a hero of the Battle of San Jacinto, who would soon be elected president of the Republic of Texas. Using his name ensured immediate recognition that the brothers hoped would entice officials to locate the new seat of government in this fledging community. They immediately began to advertise their city as a pleasantly situated place of great potential for success and business opportunity. Just four months after Texans secured their independence at San Jacinto, an advertisement published in the *Telegraph & Texas Register,* August 30, 1836, and soon circulated throughout much of Europe, promoted this notion, boldly stating: "There is no place in Texas more healthy, having an abundance of excellent spring water, and enjoying the sea breeze in all its freshness."[1]

The struggling town on Buffalo Bayou served as the capital of the Republic of Texas from 1836 to 1839 and quickly attracted its share of entrepreneurs and rapscallions, dreamers and visionaries, tradesmen and farmers, and all manner of folk looking for a fresh start in the new nation precariously positioned at the edge of both the US and Mexican frontiers. One key to the success of both the young frontier republic and its crude, temporary capital on Buffalo Bayou was the role of physicians who arrived with dreams and ambitions of their own. The grim reality of what all of these people found upon their arrival stood in stark contrast to the *Telegraph & Texas Register* advertisement, which promised a "handsome and beautifully elevated, salubrious and well watered" town site. Instead, new arrivals found the area to be flat, with dusty streets that turned quickly into a muddy quagmire after the frequent tropical rains. The conglomeration of shacks and cabins sprang up on land that was infested with mosquitoes, inhabited by alligators and snakes, and for a time nearly overrun by an overabundance of rats. Epidemics of disease and other health problems related to poor sanitation seemed at times to challenge the very survival of the community. But it was in this milieu that daring entrepreneurs found opportunity, dedicated physicians found a calling, and public health became one of the major and enduring themes deeply rooted in Houston's history. These doctors and civic leaders established a pattern that would be emulated by succeeding generations, resulting in the founding of what would in time grow into the largest medical center in the world.

Throughout Texas' history, physicians have taken major roles as leaders in government, the military, and in the community. During the Texas war for independence from Mexico, Mexican president Gen. Antonio Lopez de Santa Anna first arrived at San Antonio in February 1836 and laid siege to the Alamo. Seven of its defenders were surgeons, and only one, Dr. John Sutherland, would survive. After being injured on a scouting mission, he was dispatched to Gonzales to encourage volunteers to help defend the doomed fort. His injury saved his life. When Texans formally declared independence from Mexico on March 2, 1836, at Washington-on-the-Brazos, eight of the fifty-nine signers of the Texas Declaration of Independence were doctors. One of these physicians, Dr. Lorenzo de Zavala was chosen to be the interim vice president of the Texas government. De Zavala previously had a distinguished political career in Mexico, but resigned his post as minister to France after becoming disillusioned with Santa Anna. He moved to Texas in 1835 and purchased land along Buffalo Bayou, directly across from a place known as San Jacinto. In the aftermath of the climactic battle that took place there, his home served as a hospital for wounded Texans and Mexicans. One of the most famous surgeons in early Texas history is Dr. Anson Jones. He arrived in Texas in 1833 and, after the fall of the Alamo, joined the Texas army. He served as a surgeon at the Battle of San Jacinto and later became very active politically. After a stint as ambassador to Washington and as a representative in the Texas Congress, Jones was elected Texas' fourth and last president in September 1844. He had the distinction of presiding over annexation to the United States in February 1846.[2]

After San Jacinto, a number of doctors who served in the Texas army or in government settled in Houston—enough, in fact, to form, in 1838, a short-lived professional association, the Medical and Surgical Society of Houston. Among these early leaders was Dr. Alexander Ewing, who had been surgeon general of the Texas army at the Battle of San Jacinto, and Dr. Ashbel Smith, educated at Yale, Harvard, and in Paris and described as "physician, surgeon, statesman, and scholar." He succeeded Ewing as surgeon general and would serve as minister to France and England and as the Republic of Texas' last secretary of state. Other physicians of note include Dr. Phillip Anderson, who was chief surgeon of the Texas Navy and considered to be among the most learned men in Texas, and Dr. Francis Moore Jr., who had served in the Texas army, become editor of the *Telegraph*, and served several terms as mayor of Houston. As Houston continued to develop and evolve as a community during the 1840s, a new generation of young, well-trained doctors migrated to the town to provide medical care.[3]

Despite the ads describing Houston as a place of cool sea breezes and having a pleasant, healthy climate, the stark reality was that neither the environment nor the lifestyles and habits of its residents were conducive to good public health. Walter H. Moursund, in his study *Medicine in Greater Houston: 1836–1956*, observed that the early settlers had little knowledge of proper sanitation and hygiene and consequently became "the victims of frequent and fatal epidemics including yellow fever, malaria, dengue, typhoid, small pox, and the plague." Because they did not understand fully what caused these deadly diseases, they were unable to take proper preventive measures. The unsanitary conditions provided a better environment for rats than for people, and by early 1839 swarms of rats threatened to overrun the burgeoning community. Although early Houstonians did not yet recognize the connection between rats and the spread of typhus or the plague, on February 26, 1839, they took decisive action when John W. Eldridge organized the Anti-Rat Society with the goal of destroying the pesky infestation. And in an important second step toward cleaning up their town, in May 1839 the Houston City Council appointed the first regular Board of Health to improve sanitation and reduce the incidence of disease fostered by the filthy conditions in much of the community.[4]

As in most communities at this time, it was an uphill struggle.

Houston's first yellow fever epidemic wiped out approximately 10 percent of the population. With just 2,000 residents, the loss of some 240 during 1839, most due to the epidemic, had a sobering effect. But Houston quickly bounced back, and thus it was with jubilation that, just four years later, an article in the August 29, 1843, edition of the *Morning Star* proclaimed that with fewer cases of summer illnesses than ever before in the young community's history, the city was "remarkably healthy." The article encouraged residents to continue taking "proper precautions" in order that they might escape the diseases that frequently appeared during the warm months of summer and early fall. The editorial also noted that "fevers" seemed to become more common due to the excitement surrounding the September elections. "We hope all will bear this in mind, and endeavor to avoid all unnecessary excitement; neither giving way to passion nor intemperance." But just weeks later, during the fall of 1843, disaster again hit the city with another outbreak of yellow fever. The frightening epidemics struck the town repeatedly between 1847 and 1867.[5]

During the mid-1840s, Houston was described as a cross between a frontier town and the Wild West. One foreign visitor during this time, Prince Solms-Braunfels of Germany, commented that "Houston . . . has more houses than citizens. . . . Farmers bring their cotton here and sell it to the native businessmen, . . . Otherwise it would be only a gathering place for loafers . . . who go there mainly to gamble and trade horses with the hope of defrauding someone." Such observations aside, there were people who believed in the Allen brothers' dream, and they gambled on making Houston a major and profitable economic center. Before the outbreak of the Civil War, some of these individuals clearly had succeeded, because a number of very prosperous merchants called Houston home. The 1860 census provided not only the names of these wealthy men but revealed their net worth: for example, William Marsh Rice was worth $750,000 (about $21 million in 2011); William J. Hutchins, $700,000; Thomas William House, $500,000; Cornelius Ennis and Paul Bremond, $400,000 each (about $11.2 million in 2011)—multimillionaires today. Although they were just a few of the most prominent Houstonians at the time, their relatively early success indicated that Houston offered remarkable economic opportunities for determined entrepreneurs.[6]

Historically speaking, these men were in the right place at the right time. A growing town needed mercantile stores of every type to supply medicine, dry goods, baked goods, and clothing. It is not surprising then that this early commerce led to the success of many Houstonians, providing them with funds and opportunities to launch themselves into other business ventures. Their individual stories reveal this circle of business, trade, and investment in Houston's developing infrastructure. Col. Cornelius Ennis, mentioned above, was one of the first cotton merchants and growers in the area and exemplified this economic exchange. His success in business propelled him into taking a leadership role in the community, which led to his election as mayor of Houston in 1856. Most importantly, as one of the largest cotton buyers in Texas, Ennis fully acknowledged the opportunity cotton provided for Houston as a magnet for commerce. Moving to Houston in 1839, he had opened a drugstore, partnering with George W. Kimball. Two years later, in 1841, they sent the first cotton shipment from Galveston to Boston. Ennis quickly discovered, however, that his cotton-export business was hampered by inadequate transportation. This drove him to promote and support railroad construction in the Houston area, where he would become a strong advocate for the railroad industry. In 1853, along with Paul Bremond, William M. Rice, and Thomas W. House, Ennis began planning to incorporate the Houston and Texas Central Railroad.[7]

Thomas W. House, an Englishman, had arrived in Houston a year before Ennis in 1838. He opened a bakery, Loveridge & House, on Main Street, where two years later he and his business partner, Charles Shearn, offered ice cream and lemonade in addition to a vast assortment of baked goods. By the early 1850s, House, by then a dry goods merchant, purchased James H. Stevens and Company for $40,000, making him the largest wholesaler in the entire state. Soon after, he became one of the wealthiest landowners in Texas. As a cotton grower and factor, House was very active in the affairs of Houston's economy, maintaining several diverse roles and devoting many years of service to establishing Houston as a major economic center. As treasurer of the Houston Cotton Exchange, he became involved in the operations of the Buffalo Bayou Ship Channel Company while organizing the Houston and Galveston Navigation Company in 1851. Although he operated as a private banker, as many businessmen did in those days, he also played a substantial role in Houston's structural development by reinvesting his business profits into the region's railroads and the city's public utilities. Acknowledging very early on that both accessibility and infrastructure were important elements for the city's economic growth, men such as Ennis and House embraced the need for railroads and the development of a deepwater port. By doing so, they provided significant leadership, guidance, and much-needed capital for the advancement of Houston's status to the forefront as a major economic hub in Texas.[8]

As indicated by the wealth of the city's merchants, Houston slowly became a community of enterprising and successful businessmen who recognized an opportunity when it presented itself. Although cotton would come to play a predominant role in this economic prosperity, it was the region's abundance of other natural resources, as loudly touted by the Allen brothers, that provided the city with its initial economic foundation. The close proximity to the state's forests of longleaf pine, hardwoods, and cypress, for example, led to Houston's reputation as an excellent location for lumber companies and mill owners to set up their headquarters. As a result, the developing city rapidly became a major lumber center, providing an important commodity for the construction of all buildings within the region. Houston's first lumber mill, situated on Milam Street where it meets Buffalo Bayou, was constructed in the 1840s. As a lucrative business opportunity, lumber soon attracted many new residents into the city, including the Bering brothers, who moved to Houston in 1846. By 1853, they had established themselves as some of the largest lumber dealers in the city.[9]

Houston's population grew rapidly during the first couple of years after its founding, and then for almost a decade its numbers remained stagnant. In the 1840s the population actually declined after some residents moved to Austin, the newly declared capital. The city's population more than doubled between 1850 and 1858, however, and by then approximately 4,800 residents called it home. Many thought that part of the reason for Houston's thin population stemmed from the poor and inaccessible roads that led into the city. Roads were frequently flooded or difficult to maneuver. In rainy weather they were impassable, even with a team of oxen, making the cost of transporting freight extremely high and leading to exorbitant prices for even general merchandise. Texans and, most importantly, Houstonians recognized the need for good

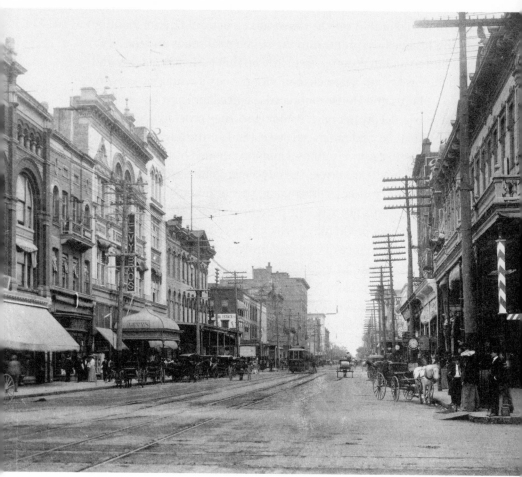

*Downtown Houston, ca. 1868. MSS-157-2535, Houston Metropolitan Research Center, Houston Public Library.*

overland transportation, and railroads seemed a likely remedy to solve the problem.[10]

Efficient transportation of cotton via railroad meant a stronger economy, and it also contributed to significant population growth as more people moved to Houston in search of employment. In these early decades, the cotton business in the city was mostly confined to the north side of Buffalo Bayou, and since there were no bridges across the bayou, the product was ferried across to the foot of Main Street. Like Ennis, however, many Houstonians looked to cotton as the potential source of

Table 1.1. Population Growth in Houston by Decade, 1850–1920

| Year | Population | Growth Percentage |
|------|-----------|-------------------|
| 1850 | 2,396 | |
| 1860 | 4,845 | 102 |
| 1870 | 9,332 | 93.6 |
| 1880 | 16,513 | 76 |
| 1890 | 27,557 | 67 |
| 1900 | 44,633 | 61.9 |
| 1910 | 78,800 | 76.5 |
| 1920 | 138,276 | 75.5 |

Source: *U.S. Census of Population, 1850–1960*. Reprinted from Marvin Hurley, *Decisive Years for Houston* (Houston: Houston Chamber of Commerce, 1966), 415.

their own individual wealth and as the key to the economic strength, stability, and prosperity of the entire region. Houstonians were thus linked to the cotton industry in a variety of ways, and it figured into the livelihood of many residents. As early as 1845, the Houston City Council viewed cotton production as so important that it passed a resolution requiring the cotton market master to report the weekly cotton sales and exports. While some cotton was transported overland by wagons, many cotton planters chose to ship their cotton by steamboats, keelboats, or flatboats. Indeed, most of the cargo moving along Buffalo Bayou by 1849 was cotton.[11]

Houston's railroad promoters understood the importance of good communication and transportation networks, and a number of these were the same influential businessmen who made a notable income from cotton. Cotton, in fact, became the impetus for the very first railroad in Texas, the Buffalo Bayou, Brazos, and Colorado Railway, which opened in 1853 with service from Harrisburg to Stafford's Point. While it was sometimes referred to as the Harrisburg Railroad, Houston equally benefited from its service. Indeed, such railroad construction translated into consequential advantages for many Houstonians. As railroad operations expanded, land values in the Houston area increased, further stimulating the economy.[12]

Cotton would come to dominate Houston's early business activity: the growing, the processing, and the transporting of the crop all took place within the area, facilitated through an emerging infrastructure of banking and improved transportation. As railroad construction continued, more land was dedicated to cotton farming, especially the vast regions to the north and west of Houston. Cotton grown there, and in other regions such as the lower Rio Grande Valley, Black Waxy Prairie, upper Rio Grande Valley, and the Texas High Plains, for example, was shipped to Houston and then on to the eastern United States and eventually to European ports. Cotton exports increased fourfold during the 1850s, thus establishing the dominance of the cotton industry as a catalyst for even more railroad construction. Clearly, Houston's emerging railroads were essential in this transportation flow, but the need for the city to develop dependable water transportation for the efficient export of this bulky crop would soon play a prominent role in the thinking of Houston's business leaders.[13]

With the city as the headquarters for many railroad, cotton, and lumber companies, Houston thus gained an enormous economic advantage in the struggle to supersede Galveston as the region's dominant center. Until oil was later discovered at nearby Spindletop at the turn of the century, at least two-thirds of Houston's economic base was linked to the transportation of natural resources such as lumber, cattle, grain, and, of course, cotton. Tremendous quantities of cotton were shipped to the city; in 1858, for example, a local newspaper reported a record cotton shipment to Houston of 522 bales, which took nineteen train cars to transport. Cotton as a basis for Houston's economic preeminence would reach a peak in the 1880s, when demands for cotton in the industrialized world increased.[14]

Since cotton was the region's main export, solving the transportation issue remained a top priority. Railroads solved only part of the problem, however, and did not remedy the dilemma of efficient, effective, and inexpensive transportation of cotton to the East Coast or to Europe. Cotton's bulkiness was clearly a factor, since it required cheaper and more efficient water transportation. In time, Houston's city boosters and businessmen would promote and put forward the idea of a ship channel as a means of gaining all-important access to transportation by sea. Although there was much to be done to secure Houston's place as an economic hub for the new century, the Allen brothers' proclamation of a city rich with resources and land was becoming more a reality than even they could have envisioned in 1836. Houston was a city full of opportunities, and cotton would continue to play a dominant role in the lives of many who succeeded financially. Cotton offered many individuals the means to make the dream of economic success come true as long as they had a little ingenuity, drive, and courage.[15]

The very same men who were instrumental in bringing the railroads to Houston assisted with ushering in the Port of Houston and developing the Houston Ship Channel. The Houston Navigation Company had been organized in 1851 by Houston merchants William Marsh Rice, Cornelius Ennis, and Paul Bremond, along with several steamboat captains, including Capt. John H. Sterrett. During the 1850s, the company dominated shipping on Buffalo Bayou, operating three steamboats that moved goods from Houston to Galveston, with the bulk of their cargo being cotton. During this early period, tariff rates were still considered reasonable: fifty cents for a bale of cotton. By the end of the decade, however, the Galveston Wharf Company increased the tariffs and also began charging excessive wharfage fees. These actions caused many Houston businessmen and ship captains to investigate new ways to bypass shipping their goods to Galveston. The major cotton interests suggested pressing cotton in Houston instead of at Galveston and shipping cotton by barges from Buffalo Bayou to the ocean vessels in Galveston Bay. In the end, they became advocates of lightering, a method of shipping goods by barge and then unloading or loading materials from larger ocean vessels onto or off the barges. This tactic became extremely popular and continued until the outbreak of the Civil War.[16]

Although Houston and most of Texas were not exposed to as much of the war's destruction as the rest of the South, the Civil War did leave its scars on the area in other ways. After the conflict, many of the railroads responsible for transporting goods and cotton to Houston were in disrepair, and even Buffalo Bayou suffered severely from years of neglect. The areas along the bayou close to Houston were especially in bad shape, with numerous snags, well-formed shoals, and the reappearance of unmaintained sandbars that interfered with shipping. By war's end, however, Houston businessmen were eager to get back to business. With that at the forefront, the Houston City Council, along with some of the Houston Cotton Exchange members, Mayor Horace Taylor and banker T. M. Bagby, and some familiar local businessmen such as William Marsh Rice and Capt. John H. Sterrett, organized the Houston Direct Navigation Company. Their immediate objective was reinstituting mid-channel lightering to bypass the Galveston Wharf Company and its exorbitant fees. The Houston Direct Navigation Company quickly achieved great success with regards to lightering. Between the years 1869 and 1881, the company alone shipped 1,985,806 bales of cotton down Buffalo Bayou. Shipping cotton still remained extremely difficult, however, due to the product's bulkiness. The members of the Houston Cotton Exchange saw the inefficiency of lightering and recognized that Houston needed a ship channel and a deepwater port if the problems of transportation were to be truly resolved.[17]

One such member was George W. Kidd, the pioneer secretary of the Houston Cotton Exchange. He supported the construction of a ship channel by gathering important data and passing it along to other like-minded boosters of the project, including Mayor Horace Baldwin Rice, H. W. Garrow, president of the Houston Cotton Exchange, and R. D. Gribble, president of the Houston Business League. Among the data submitted by these men to the US Army Corps of Engineers was the staggering figure of 5,986,437 bales of cotton, in total, transported down Buffalo Bayou between January 1, 1869, and July 8, 1897. As it turns out, the information they gathered would prove instrumental in the Corps' final approval for the Buffalo Bayou project, leading directly to the early phases of the Houston Ship Channel.[18]

Houston bankers, cotton trade members, and other businessmen similarily maintained very close relationships regarding the development of the Houston Ship Channel. Such alliances continued to develop as these business leaders worked to improve commerce in Houston. As noted above, the Houston Board of Trade and Cotton Exchange, established in 1874, was equally involved in the process (the name was changed in an 1877 charter to the Houston Cotton Exchange and Board of Trade). Although the exchange's primary goal was to regulate and organize the cotton trade, the shipping problems related to cotton's bulkiness remained one of its chief business concerns. Inexpensive and efficient water transportation was at the top of the list, since the cotton shipments were mainly for foreign markets. The organization became a strong advocate for developing the ship channel. Many of its members lobbied the federal government for aid and assistance for the ship channel as well. As cotton production expanded in the region, the US government could not ignore the profitability of the product and the increasingly vociferous solicitations from Houston's cotton interests.[19]

By the 1880s, many cotton farmers were extremely successful and wealthy, and this in turn attracted more cotton merchants and businesses to the area. In 1882 Texas produced the greatest cotton crop in history. As a result, a phenomenal amount of the cotton crop was transported into Houston, stressing the warehouse and storage facilities as never before. More than seven million bales of cotton came into the city that year, which led to the addition of two more compresses and new warehouses. Houstonians boasted that they had the largest cottonseed mills and the largest cottonseed production in the world. Indeed, by 1897, Houston was second only to New Orleans as a leading market for the purchase of cotton in the United States, and thirty-three cotton firms maintained their offices in the city.[20] While the growth in the cotton industry seemed insuppressible, so too was Houston's population. By 1900, the city still only had 5 percent of the entire region's population, but it had surpassed its nearest competitor, Galveston. Houston's population was reported to be between 40,000 and 50,000, or about one-sixth the size of New Orleans and the same size as Yonkers, New York, and Norfolk, Virginia, at that time. Furthermore, as the turn of the century neared on New Year's Eve, 1899, Houston maintained the largest railroad center south of St. Louis. With its growing reputation as a transportation hub, the Army Corps of Engineers finally agreed with the need for a ship channel and accepted the suggestions of Houston's ship channel advocates. Houstonians were closer than ever to achieving their goal of a deepwater port and a ship channel.[21]

During these years of economic development and population growth, doctors in Houston strived to improve their professional capabilities and find new ways to improve public health in the community. They formed a succession of professional organizations, beginning with the short-lived Medical and Surgical Society of Houston. In March 1857 doctors established the Houston Medical Association, "To cultivate the science of medicine and all its collateral branches; to cherish and sustain medical character; to encourage medical etiquette and to promote mutual improvement, social intercourse, and good feeling among members of the profession." The organization came to an end during the years of the Civil War. Following the war, in 1868, Houston-area physicians established the Harris County Medical Association, but that organization soon disappeared as well. The attempts to create a lasting professional association proved unsuccessful until 1894, when doctors formed the Houston District Medical Association. This group stayed together and then reorganized on July 27, 1903, with sixty-five members, to form the Harris County Medical Society (HCMS). The new medical society soon scored a major victory when, in 1907, members successfully lobbied state officials to create the Texas State Board of Medical Examiners, which established the first standards for education, training, and licensing of Texas physicians. Throughout its history, HCMS members have endeavored to raise medical standards and improve health care in Harris County.[22]

Even as Houston's population continued to grow during the nineteenth century, so too did attempts to provide improved medical care and hospitals. Evidence suggests that the first hospital to appear in Houston was a temporary facility that the Congress of the Republic of Texas authorized in October 1837 to provide care for sick soldiers. An 1839 reference in the *Morning Star* mentioned "City Hospital," and the *Weekly Telegraph* published a report in 1856 by one Henry Vanderlinden, who was identified as "Chief Clerk" of the Charity Hospital. Local doctors often teamed up in their efforts to establish hospitals, but generally these attempts were quite rudimentary. It is interesting to note the humble beginnings of hospital care in Houston in order to track the degree of change over time, from what some described as "pest houses" to an age when the city claimed some of the finest hospitals in the world.[23]

Medical care continued to evolve slowly during the late nineteenth century, with most people seeking treatment from their family doctor and long-term care from their families. Dr. David F. Stuart arrived in Houston sometime in 1867, in time both to contract and then to survive a bout of yellow fever during the epidemic of that year. During the early 1870s, Stuart and Dr. Joshua Larendon, who had served as Houston's health officer, established the city's first railroad hospital, the Houston

Infirmary. Railroads sponsored hospitals in many cities across the country, including Houston. The doctors operated the hospital on a contract basis. Dr. T. J. Boyles later joined Stuart in a second contract that included providing food and shelter along with medical care. Although details are sketchy, evidence indicates that by 1883 county commissioners had taken ownership of a cluster of frame buildings on Washington Avenue that were known variously in the community by several names, including Charity Hospital, County Hospital, the Poor House, and the Stuart and Boyles Infirmary. In his study of early medical care in Houston, Dr. Walter H. Moursund wrote that this hospital was moved to a location closer to the railroad. Apparently, it experienced many problems under Stuart and Boyles, including allegations that some patients had to wait on each other and that others slept on the floor to save costs, which further tarnished the hospital's reputation. Moursund noted that despite the many challenges they faced, before their contract expired in 1889, Stuart and Boyles were credited with establishing a program for training interns—possibly the first medical training program in Houston. Information is tentative, but it appears that the hospital continued to provide some services until it finally closed its doors in 1913.[24]

One of the most significant developments in hospital care in Houston during the late nineteenth century occurred on June 7, 1887, when six nuns from the Sisters of Charity of the Incarnate Word arrived from St. Mary's Infirmary in Galveston to establish St. Joseph's Infirmary. The sisters opened their forty-bed hospital in a frame building at Franklin and Caroline Streets. In 1889 they added a second building, enabling them to provide charity health care for the indigent. To meet Houston's growing need for hospital care, in 1893 they built a three-story brick building on Franklin Street with room for seventy-five beds. About one year later, on October 16, 1894, fire consumed all four buildings. The Sisters asked for help from the public to build another hospital, and Houstonians responded enthusiastically. The Sisters raised enough money to purchase the block between Crawford and LaBranch and bounded by Pierce and Calhoun Streets (St. Joseph's Parkway today), and constructed a 100-bed hospital, which opened in March 1896. In 1905 the hospital added a three-story brick wing and also opened the St. Joseph's Infirmary Training School for Nurses with an initial class of five students. Both the hospital and nursing program continued to grow during the ensuing years. Today St. Joseph's Hospital is the only one of Houston's downtown hospitals to survive in its downtown location into the twenty-first century.[25]

For reasons not clear, 1907 proved to be an active year for starting hospitals in Houston. In May 1907, Drs. J. H. Sampson, J. Allen Kyle, and W. A. Stevens opened the Physician's and Surgeon's Hospital Company of Houston on Calhoun Avenue, and during the same month the Salvation Army offered free services from a team of volunteers that included Dr. A. Philo Howard. Two months later, in July 1907, Drs. Haley and Barrell opened a sanitarium at 811 Main Street to provide surgery and treat general diseases. Their hospital survived only a few months; on February 28, 1908, they closed its doors and moved their equipment to the Baptist Sanitarium (formerly the Rudisill Sanitarium).[26]

The first mention of the Rudisill Sanitarium (forerunner of Memorial Hospital, known today as the Memorial Hermann Healthcare System) appeared in the *Texas State Journal of Medicine* in December 1905, when Mrs. Ida J. Rudisill moved her sanitarium into a new facility on the corner of Smith Street and Lamar Avenue. The twenty-two-bed hospital claimed "the best modern equipment for the treatment of disease" along with bathrooms, a sterilizing room, and operating rooms. On August 6, 1907, Rudisill sold her sanitarium for $18,000 to a board of trustees organized by two local Baptist ministers, Dr. L. T. Mays, pastor of the Tuam Avenue Church, and Reverend D. R. Peveto, assistant pastor of the First Baptist Church. The hospital reorganized as a charity hospital, the Baptist Sanitarium, with a medical staff that included Dr. W. W. Ralston as chairman and Dr. Oscar L. Norsworthy, general surgeon. Ida Rudisill remained involved in health care and chartered one of the first nursing schools in Houston in 1907, apparently not long after selling her hospital. The Baptist Sanitarium Hospital Training School later became the Baptist Hospital School of Nursing and then the Memorial Hospital School of Nursing. In 1911 the Baptist Sanitarium constructed a four-story addition to the back of the original building, increasing the capacity to fifty beds. More construction enlarged the hospital to a 100-bed capacity in 1915, and in 1922 the name changed to Baptist Hospital. Following demolition of the original frame structure in 1923, a new seven-story building increased capacity to 215 beds. Interestingly, in 1908, Norsworthy had opened a thirty-bed hospital on

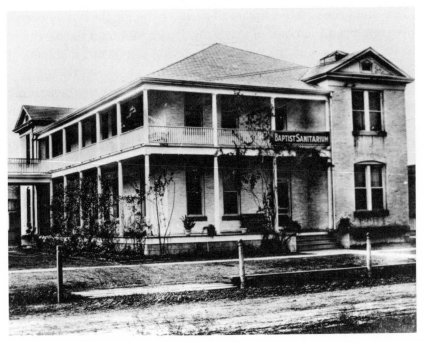

*Baptist Sanitarium, ca. 1908, forerunner to Memorial Hospital. John P. McGovern Historical Collections and Research Center, Texas Medical Center Library.*

San Jacinto at Rosalie. The Texas Conference of the Methodist Episcopal Church–South took ownership of the Norsworthy Hospital on December 31, 1919, and in it established Methodist Hospital.[27]

As mentioned earlier, railroad hospitals played an important role in health care in Texas, including Houston. One of the city's earliest modern hospitals, the Southern Pacific Hospital, opened on May 27, 1911, at 2015 Thomas Street. The 102-bed, $200,000 hospital was solidly constructed of brick and masonry and offered patients luxurious mattresses along with electricity, gas, and steam heating. It was largely through the efforts of Dr. R. W. Knox, chief surgeon of the Southern Pacific Lines, that the hospital was built. The name of the facility was changed in 1913 to the Hospital Association of the Sunset Central Lines, and four years later to the Hospital Association of the Southern Pacific Lines in Texas and Louisiana. Early in 1931 a new addition increased the capacity of the hospital from 125 to 158 beds. Later, administrators made other changes to increase efficiency, including the installation of new equipment, removal of the X-ray department from the basement to the first floor, and the refurbishing of the basement for outpatient services.[28]

During the next thirty years, new hospitals opened in a continuing effort to meet the medical needs of Houston's growing population.[29] In September 1912, Dr. James Greenwood opened his sanitarium on Old South Main Street at Oak Hill. Soon joined by Drs. Marvin L. Graves and George H. Moody, the staff provided treatment for up to thirty patients for alcohol and drug addictions, nervous diseases, and some mental diseases. In 1922 two ophthalmologists, Drs. W. W. Ralston and Everett L. Goar, formed a partnership. During the next two years, they brought in Drs. John Foster, Claude C. Cody Jr., and Lyle J. Logue, and together they built the Houston Eye, Ear, Nose, and Throat Hospital, which opened in 1924 on Caroline at Walker. That same year, the city opened Jefferson Davis Hospital at 1101 Elder. The four-story, 150-bed hospital was built at a cost of $400,000 and was the first city-owned hospital to accept indigent patients. Apparently, the hospital was constructed over a Confederate burial ground, causing Houston mayor Oscar Holcombe to name the hospital after Jefferson Davis, the president of the Confederacy, in an attempt to placate a public chorus of disapproval that erupted when it became widely known where the city was erecting its new hospital. The following year, on July 1, 1925, Hermann Hospital finally opened in a location that many considered as "out in the country," about four miles south of downtown. The new hospital had its own electric light plant, ice plant, and an electric kitchen. It was considered by some to be the finest hospital "in beauty and efficiency" anywhere in the South. The Houston Negro Hospital, known today as Riverside Hospital, opened at 3204 Ennis Street in July 1927 as the first nonprofit hospital for African American patients in the city. Oilman Joseph S. Cullinan contributed $80,000 to help construct the fifty-bed hospital. Shortly thereafter, the Houston Negro Hospital Nursing School, the first institution to train African American nurses, also opened. Prior to this, in Jim Crow–era Houston, black patients had to be admitted to racially segregated wards in local hospitals. During the next fifteen years, Park View Hospital opened (1931), followed by the Wright Clinic and Hospital on North Main (1937) and the Hedgecroft Clinic and Hospital on Montrose

(1942), which began operation as a rehabilitation hospital for children and adults afflicted and crippled by diseases, including poliomyelitis.[30]

The construction of physical health facilities went hand in hand with a growing concern to implement public health policies. During the early 1900s, business leaders, the local press, and Houston's city council actively supported improved public health and disease prevention. Officials took steps to improve the quality and safety of the food and water supply and encouraged residents within the city to connect their homes to the city sewer system. In May 1907 the city's market master received authority to inspect all farm products, fruits, and vegetables peddled to individual homes, and in August 1907 the milk inspector

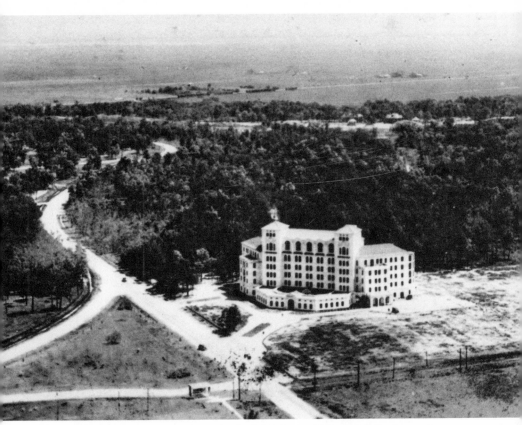

*Hermann Hospital, ca 1926. Courtesy of John P. McGovern Historical Collections and Research Center, Texas Medical Center Library.*

began analyzing milk samples from every dairy in the Houston area. Dr. George W. Larendon, the city health officer, began stricter enforcement of the ordinance against throwing trash into the waters of Buffalo Bayou in a new effort to prevent contamination of the stream. In February 1909 the Harris County Medical Society appointed a committee of three physicians, Drs. S. M. Briscoe, J. W. Scott, and J. B. York, who prepared a report for city officials that emphasized the need for a bacteriological expert to serve as pathologist for the city. Officials quickly responded and appointed Dr. Felician J. Slataper as city pathologist.[31]

By 1910, Houston's population had grown to 78,800 people. A city Health Department report the following year, dated February 28, 1911, provides a sketch of the city's public health services. The report indicated that doctors had treated 4,000 patients at the city dispensary, 550 at the hospital, thirty-six at the pest camp, and had provided vaccinations for approximately 2,000 schoolchildren. The Health Department utilized fumigation as one of its main weapons to prevent the spread of communicable diseases and had fumigated rooms, boxcars, and two autos for cerebrospinal meningitis, diphtheria, scabies, scarlet fever, smallpox, and tuberculosis. During 1911, Slataper reported that the Health Department's health laboratory conducted 1,782 microscopic and chemical examinations.[32]

As medical and public health facilities continued to expand, so too did plans for improved transportation. During these same years, the Houston committee of businessmen who organized themselves in favor of a port and the ship channel had relentlessly engaged in a campaign to convince the US Congress to appropriate the necessary funds for its development. The committee had their sights set on constructing a twenty-five-foot-deep channel from Houston to Galveston Bay. The Houston Cotton Exchange and Board of Trade assisted with this campaign by lobbying Congress for help with creating the Houston Ship Channel. Everyone agreed that water was the best way to transport huge cotton shipments, and cotton had become "the lifeblood of the Houston economy." Congress finally conceded, and the work began in earnest on the ship channel and port.[33]

By 1903, Houston's booming economy, predominately driven by cotton, secured Harris County's place as the wealthiest county in Texas.

The decision to make Houston a port city sealed the deal that Houston would be the major port for cotton shipments instead of Galveston, which recently had been devasted by the great hurricane of 1900. The next year, 1904, Houston's cotton receipts totaled 17.7 percent of all the cotton produced in the United States. The *Houston Post* reported in 1911 that Houston was the "greatest inland cotton market in the world." Cotton remained the port's most important export throughout 1913–14. When the new Houston Ship Channel finally opened on November 10, 1914, Houstonians celebrated wildly. The timing was ironic, however, since Europe was engulfed in World War I at the time, resulting in a loss of accessible markets. Furthermore, after Great Britain placed cotton on the contraband list, there was a 50 percent drop in trade for the ship channel, and the cotton market quickly collapsed. But 1917 marked the beginnings of a recovery for the market, with cotton fetching a high of $16.25 per bale. Two years later, in 1919, the economic future looked even brighter, with gross annual cotton receipts reaching 3,000,000 bales. Importantly, the federal government also approved the deepening of the Houston Ship Channel to thirty feet. In November of that year, the *Merry Mount*, loaded with 23,719 bales of cotton, became the first vessel to carry cotton directly from Houston to Europe.[34]

Throughout the 1920s, cotton remained an indispensable part of Houston's economy, its market value twice that of oil. The city became the funnel for cotton production, processing, and shipping from Arkansas, Oklahoma, Texas, and Louisiana. Local banks not only became experienced in financing cotton's expansion but were familiar with European cotton connections, too. As a result, Houston became home to more than eighty companies involved in the cotton market. The city was clearly at the forefront of the cotton industry, and the Port of Houston was continually improving, with larger warehouses, numerous cotton compresses, and channel terminals along its banks.[35]

As the city continued to grow and mature as a community, public health continued to occupy civic and medical leaders in Houston. The city Health Department remodeled its facilities in September 1919 and installed new laboratory equipment. The remodeling plans included sanitary and thoroughly modern accommodations for a new "medical clinic, a surgical clinic, an eye, ear, nose, and throat clinic, a prenatal clinic, a children's clinic, a narcotic clinic, the public health nursing department, and the offices of the physician and secretaries in charge of the health department."[36]

During the ensuing years, as Houston's economy thrived and its population continued to increase, the city served as the host for several major public health conferences, including the fifth Texas Sanitarians' Short School, November 1–4, 1927. The annual Short School returned a few years later under its new name, the Texas Public Health Association, at the Rice Hotel on November 9–14, 1931. Public health continued to be a major issue in the city during the years of the Great Depression and into the 1940s. The City Health Board, led by Dr. Frederick C. Elliott, dean of the Texas Dental College, encouraged city officials to consider obtaining a $100,000 grant from the federal government in September 1938 to establish two new health centers.[37]

The first Public Health Institute of Houston was held on December 2, 1940, at the Rice Hotel. Directors of health and social welfare in Houston coordinated their work into a preventive medicine program in 1941. Two years later, May 24–25, 1943, the Committee on Public Health of the Houston Chamber of Commerce sponsored a public health conference. Mayor Otis Massey and William Strauss, chairman of the committee, welcomed the guests to a full first day that included presentations by local physicians and public health officials. The program illustrates the diversity of subjects involved in the field of public health, as the second day was devoted to discussions of "industrial hygiene, sanitation, occupational hazards, sewage disposal and water, mosquitoes, venereal disease, and rat control . . . and prevention and control of tuberculosis." In December the Texas Public Health Association sponsored a Public Health Institute in which representatives from the city of Houston and seven county public health units participated.[38]

By this time, the state legislature had authorized the creation of a new state cancer hospital (1941) and the M. D. Anderson Foundation—created in 1936—had begun to take the leading role to establish a major medical center in the city. The trustees of the Anderson Foundation were well aware of the health needs of the city and, even more importantly, had begun to develop a broader vision for what could be accomplished in the community. Creating a medical center in Houston was a logical next step in the city's public health history. Almost from its founding in 1836, public health was one of the major concerns for Houston's civic leaders. Nearly 100 years to the date after the Allen brothers established the city, Monroe D. Anderson would create his charitable foundation with the greatest of intentions, little realizing the significant role it would have not only for improving health care for Houstonians, but also in providing the impetus to create a center that would lead the way in medical research and patient care for all of humanity. It was in this business and public health environment that the city of Houston grew as a community and continued to attract people who possessed both an entrepreneurial spirit, with its capacity to dream boldly, and a deep appreciation for the opportunities the city had offered to them. Thus, the story of the creation of the Texas Medical Center is in part the story of Houston and the environment that attracted community-minded entrepreneurs like Monroe Anderson and helped foster their success. The result is Anderson's gift to Houston, the M. D. Anderson Foundation, and in turn, Houston's gift to the world, the Texas Medical Center.

# Chapter 2

## *Building the Fortune*

### Anderson, Clayton & Company

At the turn of the twentieth century, Houston continued as a magnet for a myriad of enterprising businessmen who realized the gain to be found in lumber, cotton, and, later, oil. The individuals who came to Houston recognizing the city's economic opportunities all shared certain traits: drive, stamina, business acumen, and, most importantly, a spirit of entrepreneurship. Many of these risk-takers were adventurous men who through hard work, and sometimes extreme frugality, became wealthy and prominent Houstonians. They never forgot their origins and the struggles they endured to achieve their goals, however. For this reason, they generally gave back to society, and their philanthropy significantly influenced Houston and, in some cases, the outside world. The early history of Anderson, Clayton & Company, which in time became the world's largest cotton-trading firm, well illustrates this attitude. Later, the success of this firm enabled one of its founders, Monroe Dunaway Anderson, to achieve a spectacular level of financial success that in turn would provide the wellspring of funds and business leadership to launch the Texas Medical Center.

The company's founders, actually two pairs of brothers, were related to each other by marriage. Each of these men possessed specific talents and skills in various fields that enabled their company to reach amazing heights and eventually become a global success. As Anderson, Clayton & Company grew in physical and financial stature, the company's founders—hardworking, adventurous entrepreneurs—were catapulted to a level of unprecedented wealth. Frank Ervin Anderson and Monroe Dunaway Anderson, one pair of the firm's founding brothers, were the sons of Tennessean James Wisdom Anderson and his wife, Mary Ellen Dunaway Anderson. In 1862 James Anderson became a volunteer in the Confederate Army, but early on in his service he was captured by Union soldiers and sent to Camp Chase, a federal prison camp near Columbus, Ohio. Anderson served nearly three years there, surviving the frigid winters in unheated facilities. In 1865 he was exchanged for a Union prisoner. Upon his arrival home in Tennessee, Mary informed him that a son, William Thomas, had been born in his absence. It took no time for James and Mary to add to their brood, increasing the size of the Anderson family to eight children in all: Frank was born on July 22, 1868, while Monroe arrived in the world on June 29, 1873.[1]

Life in the ruptured and economically deprived South after the end of the Civil War taught both boys the value of a dollar. As youngsters, they became well acquainted with the demands and benefits of austerity and frugality. Although the South's economy suffered during the postwar years, banking remained relatively stable, since it was the linchpin of the South's agricultural business. More importantly, Tennessee's state leadership supported new banking ventures during this difficult, transitional period. James Anderson took the opportunity to assist with establishing the First National Bank of Jackson in 1873 and remained there as its president until 1879, when he died suddenly at the age of forty-four. Most of the Anderson children were still very young when their father died; Frank was eleven, and Monroe was only five. Although James provided Mary and the children with an income, the family's finances were hardly sufficient to support eight children. Mary encouraged the boys to take on various duties to earn additional income. These life experiences would become forever ingrained in Frank and Monroe, having a profound, lifelong influence on the way they handled their money.[2]

As young men, both Frank and Monroe attended college, but only Frank, who attended Cumberland College in Lebanon, Tennessee, actually graduated, and his exact degree is unknown. Frank was the first of the Anderson brothers to go into the banking business, working at the bank his father helped establish in Jackson. Yet Frank had different ideas about his future. As he became more and more interested in the cotton industry, he saw a future in the commodity. Since cotton continued to play a pivotal role in the South's economic recovery, Frank quickly realized that any connection with the cotton business could potentially be very successful. Accordingly, he began studying and practicing the skills necessary to inspect and judge the quality and color of raw cotton.[3]

Grading cotton was a technical skill, and good eyesight was an essential requirement for cotton classers. Frank excelled in this area and soon became an expert. He could determine the suitability of cotton for manufacturing thread and fabrics, but he was especially keen at judging its fair market value. There were several key factors that determined the value of cotton and bales of cotton: staple—the length of the fiber (to the sixteenth of an inch), grade (from pure white to off-color with some trash), and the weight of each bale (usually about 500 pounds). Good classers saw cotton differently, as each crop revealed various shades that significantly affected the overall market price. The whiter the cotton fiber, the better the grade and the higher the price it would bring at market. If the fiber was not the true or purest shade of white, it received the lower grade. Every bale had its own unique value. Baled cotton was marketed in 100-bale running lots (same grade and staple), and with the value based on grade, staple, and total weight. Warehouse receipts were issued for each bale and used as collateral for short-term bank loans needed to finance the holdings of the huge quantities of cotton bought each season and held before they were sold.[4]

Frank's astuteness enabled him to become a professional and skilled cotton merchant, buying and selling "King Cotton" for the firm of Dobbins and Daisey in Nashville, Tennessee. By 1895, he was a successful cotton buyer for George H. McFadden, a national firm headquartered in Philadelphia. It was at this time that he proposed to Dessie Burdine Clayton, and they were married in Jackson, Tennessee, on August 22, 1895. According to their son, Thomas, his mother's name, Dessie, was derived from Desdemona, a character in Shakespeare's *Othello*. Following her marriage to Frank Anderson, she dropped Dessie from her name and thereafter went by Burdine Clayton Anderson. After the wedding, Frank established a small cotton-buying company in Jackson, purchasing cotton in western Tennessee for his uncle Neil Anderson, who owned a profitable cotton firm in Fort Worth, Texas. Although Frank and Burdine lived for the next five years in Jackson, Frank's business contact with his uncle would prove fortuitous for the young couple. Neil

Anderson was a strong believer in the new Territory of Oklahoma and its promise of good cotton-growing lands. A few years earlier, in 1889, huge sections of the territory opened up to settlers who would clear much of this land by the end of the century. Many of these settlers had become cotton farmers, and Neil Anderson wanted to be part of this emerging cotton-growing region.[5]

In early 1900, Neil Anderson sent Frank on an exploratory mission to Oklahoma City, a small town at the time, with a population of around 10,000. The town had emerged as a result of the construction of the Santa Fe and Rock Island Railroads, which ran right through its center. Businesses and homes were rapidly constructed near the train crossing and in the surrounding area. After Frank reported back to his uncle, they decided it was prime time to open an office in this new, foundling city. Frank rode the Rock Island Railroad back to Oklahoma City, setting up the office to begin the process of buying and selling cotton in the name of his uncle's firm. Within a short time, the office was doing enough business that Frank decided to move Burdine and his family to Oklahoma City. Neil Anderson's prediction proved extremely accurate: the area had a significant need for individuals who were knowledgeable about raw cotton and who were ready to maximize the potential of this commodity.[6]

Although Frank respected and appreciated the opportunity his uncle had offered him, he had always dreamed of being his own boss. He knew that now was the time to make this leap and go into business on his own. In fact, as early as December 1902, correspondence indicates that Frank and Monroe Anderson were thinking seriously of going into the cotton business. On December 27, 1902, Frank wrote to Monroe from Oklahoma City, stating, "In regard to going in for ourselves next season . . . I think the opportunity for doing well out here is unequalled anywhere. It is only a question of surviving the expense of getting started, and the probability of having a bad season at the outset." Frank had decided to put down roots in Oklahoma, and in the same letter he announced that he was going to "build us a little cottage here." In January 1903, Frank began searching for partners who also recognized that this was an incredible chance for success. In a letter to Monroe, Frank hinted that he was thinking about leaving his uncle's firm, "but could not come to any final conclusion as to the matter we had under

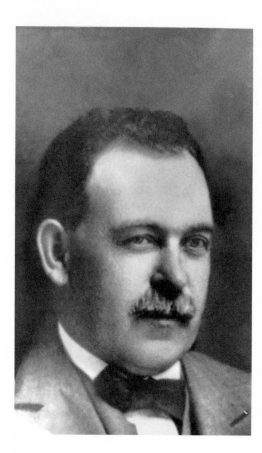

*Frank E. Anderson.*
*RG-E-61-9, Houston*
*Metropolitan Research*
*Center, Houston Public*
*Library.*

consideration." During the succeeding months, Frank and Monroe discussed the details and shared many ideas about starting their own cotton business. Frank was concerned about how much money they would need to start their own company, estimating they would need startup capital and credit of about "$25,000 to $30,000" to begin. On April 13, 1903, Frank again wrote to Monroe regarding his brother's latest proposition of starting a cotton business. "It will take a good deal of money to handle a cotton account correctly and to hedge the trades with futures when necessary," he wrote. "But I think with careful handling we ought to get along all right. It also takes a good deal more money to run a business out here than it does back there and we will have to decide between the two." Burdine understood and encouraged Frank to take advantage of the situation by offering to mortgage their home for the initial investment of $3,000. With Burdine's support, Frank's confidence in his own ability and in the cotton industry soared.[7]

Monroe Anderson had taken a different path than his older brother, Frank. After completing the eighth grade, Monroe briefly attended Southwestern Baptist University in Jackson. While he was still in college, however, another uncle, Hugh Anderson, proposed that Monroe take the position as the assistant cashier at his bank, the People's National Bank. A quick study of the banking and financing industry, Monroe took this job very seriously, greeting the clients very courteously and professionally. His friends and family regarded Monroe as a good-natured, stylish, and neatly attired young professional. And they also saw that he was, even at the early age of twenty-two, an extremely cautious banker. He maintained his position at the bank for ten years, over time obtaining the nickname of the "careful cashier." He became a student of calculated risk by determining good loans with expected interest-based paybacks by the recipients. At the same time, he began putting away money for his own future. Whenever he had a little to spare, he deposited it in the bank. By 1904, Monroe was an experienced banker, and his colleagues frequently referred to him as a financial genius. Yet the one attribute that Monroe Anderson became widely recognized for could not be taught: he was an extremely good judge of character.[8]

Monroe was still working at the Jackson bank when Frank initially approached him, explaining his latest idea for a cotton business. After several months of correspondence and discussions, Monroe accepted Frank's offer and put up $3,000 of his own savings for his share of the investment. Uncle Neil also supported the endeavor and promised assistance if needed for the venture. Frank knew from his experience with his uncle's business, however, that this initial investment was not enough. Still in need of additional funds, he and Burdine decided that New York City might offer the extra assistance they required, especially in light of the fact that Will Clayton, Burdine's brother, was an officer with the American Cotton Company in the city at the time. On June 29, 1904, Frank wrote to Monroe that he had resigned from his uncle's cotton firm. "It is now up to us to make a living for ourselves out of the cotton business," wrote Frank. "They did not express much sorrow at losing me, but said they could not blame me for wanting to go in for myself. Our hope of doing a large business I think lies in getting the assistance of Will C

[Clayton] who can command some very good correspondents, and who can also bring the A. Cot. Co. [American Cotton Company] business with him, as explained to you in my last letter." Frank prepared to rent an office and secure the necessary office supplies, and he asked Monroe to arrange a $500 loan to assist him. "This must not be neglected, but attended to at once as I will be out of funds practically by the middle of July. I can arrange a mortgage on my property here to put into the cotton account but do not wish to do so now. Let me hear from you at once."[9]

The second set of Anderson, Clayton & Company's founding brothers were also no strangers to economic struggle. William (Will) Lockhart Clayton was born on a cotton farm near Tupelo, Mississippi, on February 7, 1880. His father, James Monroe Clayton, experienced many hardships in providing for his family over the years and only barely managed financially with the help of his wife, Fletcher Burdine Clayton. Working initially as a schoolteacher, James inherited the family cotton farm after the death of his parents but soon fell deep into debt and was forced to mortgage the property to his uncle. In time, a family friend offered Clayton a job at a hardware store in Jackson, Tennessee, resulting in the family moving to the city when Will was very young. It was there that they met the Andersons. Although Fletcher Clayton ensured that her brood was neatly dressed and attended school, Will's formal education ended with the seventh grade. All too aware of the family's critical financial situation, Will began studying shorthand with a local expert as a means to earn additional income as a court reporter. At just fifteen years of age, Will became known as Jackson's speediest shorthand and typing professional. It did not take long for visiting businessmen to learn of Will and his expertise. Jerome Hill of the American Cotton Company, for example, visited Jackson frequently during this time as he checked on the development of a round bale press. Will Clayton frequently worked for Hill during this period, and soon Hill offered the young man a permanent job in St. Louis. Against his mother's wishes, he accepted the position and moved to St. Louis in 1895. After only one year, Hill offered Clayton a promotion to the New York City office. This new position offered additional responsibility with an increased salary, and the sixteen-year-old Will jumped at the opportunity, moving to Manhattan in 1896. Within just eight years he became the company treasurer.[10]

While Will Clayton climbed the corporate ladder with the American Cotton Company, his younger brother, Benjamin, also instilled with their mother's work ethic, assisted the family financially by working odd jobs in Jackson. Ben Clayton was born two and one-half years after Will, during the summer of 1882. Before he had left, Will had taught Ben stenography, and this skill kept Ben employed with a steady income to help the family and support himself. By age eighteen, Ben was in El Paso working for a railroad operations company, and it was here that he was offered a position by the general manager and chief engineer of Cananea Consolidated Copper Company. But Ben became ill with pneumonia about seven months later, and when he did return to work, at the age of twenty, it was at his brother's company, the American Cotton Company, in the Savannah, Georgia, office. Now both Clayton brothers worked in the cotton industry.[11]

Ben, however, did not have an easy go of it. While traveling for American Cotton from Savannah to New York City, he was taken ill again. This time he had to leave the train when it reached Washington, DC, and was transported immediately to a hospital for a surgery that left him with a serious streptococcus infection in his digestive tract. After recuperating, Ben returned to his job at American Cotton. As the person responsible for the division of traffic for the Houston territory, which included all of Texas and part of Oklahoma, he had a lot to keep up with. He managed a large cotton warehouse and was responsible for hiring and supervising over 300 personnel and laborers for the company. He was a skilled manager of the cotton gins because he understood how to mill, store, gin, and transport the product. Indeed, Ben's knowledge of railroads was a significant asset because it enabled him to adeptly coordinate the company's transportation needs.[12]

Both Clayton brothers were acquiring new skills and learning important aspects of the industry. While Ben was busy managing the Houston territory, Will had made important connections with very influential European contacts in the cotton business. He had also become an experienced hand at buying and selling cotton during his employment at American Cotton. His role was to learn how cotton needed to be processed and shipped from New York with the highest profit margin possible. This specific training left Will with an uncanny ability to calculate the prices for the purchase or sale of cotton quickly and extremely accurately.[13]

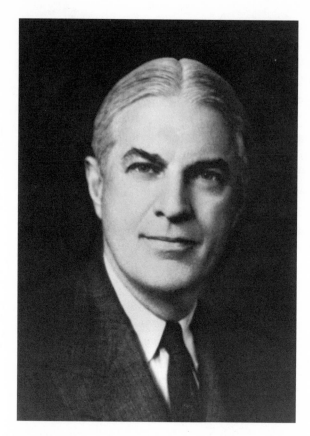

*William L. "Will" Clayton. RG-E-61-28, Houston Metropolitan Research Center, Houston Public Library.*

At the time that Frank and Burdine made their journey to New York City, Ben, at just twenty-two years of age, had been employed at the American Cotton Company for only two years. While Will had worked for the company considerably longer, he had lingering doubts about the company's sustainability and even attempted to resign at one point. His uncertainty was rooted in the company's mismanagement. Lamar Fleming Sr., general manager and Will's mentor at the company, described American Cotton as a firm that frequently overextended itself, with a top management group that did not get along and undercut each other much of the time. Yet, as discussed below, some of the company's dilemma also stemmed from the new technology of the round bale compress. While American Cotton held a patent for a round bale compress, it was not the sole owner of such a patent. In fact, one of its major competitors also had a patent for the compress. In addition to patent issues, however, the round bale compress met with an unfavorable reception from the cotton industry in the South, which still favored the square bale compress.[14]

By 1904, Will was more convinced than ever that the American Cotton Company's failure was fast approaching. Fortuitously, it was just at this time that Frank approached him with his business proposition, asking for the much-needed additional funds to kick-start his company. Keen for his brother-in-law's opportunity, Will supplied $3,000 and became a partner in Frank's new firm. He resigned as assistant general manager of American Cotton and joined Monroe and Frank Anderson to organize Anderson, Clayton & Company in August 1904. As Frank Anderson anticipated in his letter to Monroe, the American Cotton Company filed for bankruptcy later in 1904. Will Clayton was well known and highly regarded by the firm's clientele and was able to secure much of its business for the new firm. At Christmastime, Benjamin Clayton, who was still employed at American Cotton when it filed for bankruptcy, met with his brother in Fort Worth and began preparations to become the fourth member of the new firm. He officially joined the

*Benjamin Clayton.*
*RG-E-61-26, Houston*
*Metropolitan Research*
*Center, Houston Public*
*Library.*

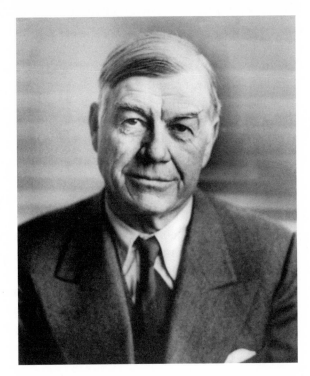

company in August 1905. So, with an investment of $3,000 from each of the four principals, Anderson, Clayton & Company was established.[15]

The ultimate success of Anderson, Clayton & Company was inextricably related to its four founding members. From the beginning, it was apparent that each of them had a substantial knowledge of the cotton industry, but each also brought individual strengths and talents. It was not just their experience or knowledge that made them successful, but the way that their skills complemented each other. Indeed, the partners' management style in those early days set the precedent for the company; each partner recognized his own strengths but also understood the synergy that came from the combination of their individual areas of expertise: Frank was an extremely skilled cotton buyer and classer; Will had developed great expertise in futures trading and cotton sales; Monroe had adept banking and money skills; and Ben was the transportation expert, extremely talented at directing warehousing and shipping.[16]

Although they were fairly young men when they established their cotton firm, the Anderson and the Clayton brothers each brought a high level of energy and enthusiasm to their fledgling business. Only thirty-six years old at the time of the company's formation, for example, Frank was very familiar with Oklahoma Territory and the cotton-growing areas of Texas. He had well-established relationships with cotton ginners, shippers, and others in the industry. He was highly regarded among these individuals as an honest, skilled, and reliable cotton grader and buyer. Monroe had an equally pristine reputation in the banking industry. At thirty-one, he had accrued ten years of wide-ranging experience dealing with merchants and farmers in the Jackson region. Cotton was the main commodity there as well, and Monroe learned to recognize a well-run operation before loaning money. Additionally, he was extremely proficient in the financial aspects of the cotton industry, using his business acumen to benefit cotton interests and his bank. Will Clayton was only twenty-four years of age at the founding of the company. No one, however, could have been better equipped with personal and professional contacts and knowledge of the product. He knew how best to transport cotton from New York to Europe, maintaining many industry contacts in various aspects of the cotton business both in the United States and in Europe. Importantly, his contacts and clients considered him a genteel and skilled negotiator. The youngest of the group, Ben Clayton, was only twenty-two years old at the time of the firm's founding. Highly respected by his employees and the individuals he dealt with daily, Ben understood how to manage clusters of cotton gins and how to coordinate the transportation of cotton from one area to another with apparent ease.[17]

Also instrumental to the early success of the company were the factors of timing and location. Frank Anderson, who had had the vision to start a cotton operation in Oklahoma, was the first to recognize that Oklahoma City was a good location to set up their firm. At the turn of the twentieth century, Oklahoma was a rapidly growing cotton area, and Anderson, Clayton & Company had entered a booming cotton industry. It was risky to open a business in Oklahoma Territory at that time, but their business focused on cotton production in the West, and most of that growth was occurring in Oklahoma and Texas. Although the firm struggled initially, the stage was set for the firm's eventual success.[18]

During this period in the United States, less than one-third of cotton growers owned their own land, with 35 percent of them being sharecroppers and 38 percent working as tenant farmers. It was a tough system, and no one had the capital to change it. The value added to cotton—buying, ginning, compressing, grading, and consolidating—were aspects handled locally, but spinning, weaving, and manufacturing of finished products were done in Europe or in New England. And at the time, New York City was the central marketing exchange for the United States, so the companies based there had a significant advantage. Cotton was actually shipped to Europe from New York, even though it would have cost far less to ship the cotton directly from Houston or from some other Southern port. This became a significant contention, since two-thirds of the US cotton crop and all of the cotton grown in Texas and Oklahoma was shipped to New York or New England before it was shipped overseas to Liverpool, Le Havre, or Bremen. Merchants in these areas stored the cotton in large warehouses, where the shipments served as collateral for the bank loans that financed the transactions until the mills were ready for delivery. Therefore, having European connections in Liverpool and the other textile regions in Europe was an essential element for a successful cotton business in the United States.[19]

The American Cotton Company had practiced large-scale speculation by buying cotton on the futures market. Cotton was a volatile commodity. Cotton merchants bought future contracts of cotton to prevent losses from unpredictable or variable pricing in a process called hedging. American Cotton went beyond this practice, attempting to make substantial profits by speculating what those futures markets might do. These speculations led to some of the company's largest losses. This had been the major reason for Will Clayton's fears about the company's future, and it had provided the impetus for his resignation. Will realized that American Cotton's top managers never completely understood that the cotton industry was changing and developing into a global enterprise in a way not seen before. But Will Clayton understood the changing market dynamics and was able to push his new company forward. The time was right for Anderson, Clayton & Company to move to the forefront of the industry and expand.[20]

From the firm's inception, therefore, the partners wanted to extend their company's reach by working directly with European contacts. To achieve this, they needed credible banking resources. Monroe remained at his banking position in Tennessee, handling the company's financial needs from afar. Although he was restricted in what resources he could provide, he was instrumental in advising and assisting with financial planning and management of the new company. In the meantime, Frank walked the fields of Oklahoma and the panhandle of Texas, looking for the best grade of cotton to fulfill the demands of their buyers. Frank's ability was widely known, as his son Thomas Anderson recalled years later: "He could walk into a field of cotton and pick a little bit out of a boll of cotton, do it like this between his fingers and say, 'strict middling, an inch a sixteenth,' or whatever it was. A very good grade." Will, meanwhile, kept up with the global market, looking for pitfalls, shortfalls, and new outlets. His knowledge of foreign markets had evolved tremendously during his employment at American Cotton. He began contacting his old European connections by traveling to Europe during the first two years of the firm's founding. These trips proved to be extremely successful endeavors in which he reestablished several of his previous relationships, enabling Anderson, Clayton & Company to profitably compete in the international cotton market. After Ben joined the company in 1905, his role was to establish and buy the local facilities for ginning, compressing, and warehousing cotton as well as the refineries for processing cottonseed into oils and feed products. Ben Clayton described Oklahoma in those early years as a remarkably rough country with few roads, poor travel, and very few accommodations for travelers. Ben's position required that he manage the thirty-six cotton gins owned by the company throughout Oklahoma and Texas. The company bought cotton in bulk from the farmers and then ginned, baled, and shipped it. He traveled throughout the area, keeping up with the process while establishing optimum shipping methods for the product.[21]

By the end of its first year in business, Anderson, Clayton & Company had handled 30,000 bales of cotton and earned a profit of about $10,000. During the next two years, this margin improved to about $60,000 each year.[22] Cotton was affecting the growth of not only the rural farm areas of Oklahoma and Texas but, at the time of the founding of Anderson, Clayton & Company, Houston's soaring cotton market, too. In 1904 cotton receipts in Houston totaled 17.7 percent of the total cotton production in the United States. Twenty years earlier the Houston Cotton Exchange and Board of Trade had constructed a building of its own on the west corner of Travis and Franklin Streets in downtown Houston. Now it was rapidly outgrowing that facility. The discovery of oil at Spindletop at the turn of the century spurred the economic development of Houston and its surrounding region with a tremendous oil boom. As the Port of Houston was gradually constructed and with over seventeen railroad lines leading into the city's center, companies that relied upon transportation for their business found that Houston was a logical choice to set up their headquarters. Houston banks, fat on the profits of oil, cotton, and lumber enterprises, were solvent and able to assist business ventures with much-needed loans. It was only a matter of time before the Anderson and Clayton brothers recognized that in Houston lay the destiny and future success of their venture.[23]

By 1907, Anderson, Clayton & Company had grown significantly and needed access to larger short-term loans and lines of credit that the limited resources of the banks in Jackson could not provide. The business had grown to the extent that it was time for Monroe Anderson to leave Jackson and devote all his time to handling the financial affairs and banking needs of Anderson, Clayton & Company. The partners decided that Houston, as a growing transportation and financial center, was a rational choice for their overall needs. They agreed that Monroe should move to the city to secure financial relations and establish a base office in anticipation of the company's eventual move.[24]

When Monroe Anderson arrived in Houston in 1907, the city had a population of about 78,000. Although there were suburbs, the majority of Houstonians lived within the city center radiating out from Main Street and Texas Avenue. There were a number of banking facilities, including the Union National Bank, the Lumbermen's National Bank, and Banker's Trust, with Jesse Jones as its chairman. Anderson acquired an office and warehouse for the firm at the foot of Bremond Street and hired B. M. Fox as his agent, changing the next year to James A. Martin, who maintained an office in the Houston Cotton Exchange building. As the company's manager for Houston, Monroe secured his own office in the Cotton Exchange building, room 208, a couple of years later. Initially, he found living quarters at the Corona Furnished Rooms facility on Walker Street.[25] In 1911 he moved to Mrs. Alice Joiner's boardinghouse at 818 Austin Street, a more prominent neighborhood featuring many beautiful, stately homes where several influential members of Houston society resided. For a time, however, it seemed that Monroe was very unhappy about living in Houston, and evidence suggests that he may have considered leaving the firm to return home to Jackson. Perhaps it was the purchase of his first car some months later that improved his outlook on life in Houston.[26]

There is no doubt that during this time Houston was a place of lively, perpetual growth and development. A sure sign of this progress and prosperity was the more frequent use of the automobile, and Monroe Anderson, like many of his contemporaries, became fascinated with the idea of owning his own car. This desire did not come from the need for transportation, since he was within walking distance of work, eateries, or anything else he might require. Nevertheless, in 1912, Monroe Anderson, the frugal banker, departed from his usual thrifty nature and purchased his first car, a four-cylinder Cadillac. Cadillacs were very expensive vehicles, but they would become a passion for Anderson, and while he owned only four cars in his lifetime, all of them were Cadillacs.[27]

Family and friends knew Monroe as a practical joker who relished harmless pranks. To others, he appeared so mild-mannered that he

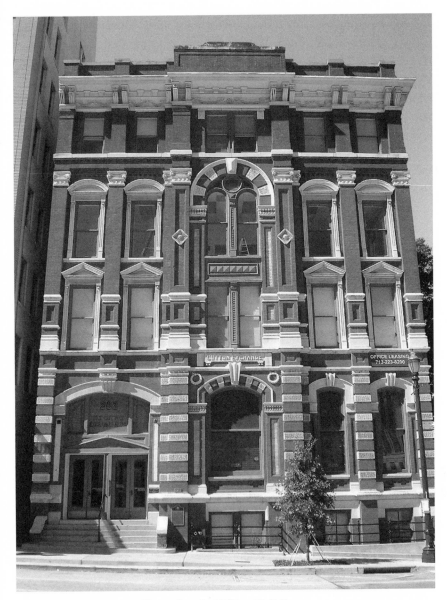

*Old Cotton Exchange Building. Photo by William H. Kellar.*

frequently surprised his victims with these jokes, since they were unaware of this tendency. He often kept on his person items such as doctored candies, hand shockers, and bogus money. Yet it was his penchant for carrying out large, well-planned schemes that many of his friends and acquaintances long remembered. No one was safe from his antics, not even the women he dated. On one such occasion, he told a date that his new car would not go forward, and he proceeded to drive around the block twice in reverse. She became so upset with him that she jumped out of the car and never saw him again. Another time, Anderson instructed his secretary to invite six couples to dinner at a very prestigious home in Houston. When the party arrived at the home, the hostess appeared at the front door in her housecoat. Everyone was quite embarrassed, and amid the stammering, red faces, and apologies appeared Monroe. With his usual good humor, he then ushered away all of his victims to an elaborate dinner on a moored passenger liner in the Turning Basin at the Port of Houston.[28]

Not being much in the way of an athlete and even somewhat against the idea of exercise, Monroe nonetheless loved to hunt and fish. He became very good friends with the company's lawyers, John H. Freeman and Col. William B. Bates. In particular, Bates and Anderson went on fishing trips together as often as they could get away.[29] And as treasurer of Anderson, Clayton & Company, Monroe became acquainted with many bankers and businessmen, some of whom became steadfast friends. He met Clarence Malone, the head of the Guardian Trust Company, in 1908, for example. Anderson held a stock interest in the bank, and over the years he and Malone became good friends. Monroe also had stock in the National Bank of Commerce in Houston and became acquainted with banker Arthur Fisher, who in turn became a dear friend. He frequently accompanied his nephews on trips to Galveston and often visited his brother's family lake house in Minnesota to partake in fishing. Although he enjoyed traveling within the United States, Monroe had never traveled out of the country until a colleague, Lamar Fleming Jr. (later to become president of Anderson, Clayton), and his wife, Clare, convinced him to go overseas on a European vacation with them. Lamar was the son of Lamar Fleming Sr., Will Clayton's mentor from his earlier days at the American Cotton Company. Monroe, as it turns out, had an excellent time, since Lamar Jr. was also a practical joker. Family stories relay how the two of them played jokes on each other for the entire duration of the trip.[30]

In a myriad of ways, Monroe D. Anderson was truly a generous person. His compassion for people down on their luck and for mankind in general can be seen in many of his actions throughout his life and likely stems, at least in part, from his family's financial struggles after his father's death. When a person came to him in need of a loan, for example, he usually sent them to the bank. Unbeknownst to the individual, however, Monroe would have called the banker, apprising him of the situation, which allowed the individual to secure the necessary funds while also keeping his dignity. Monroe did not necessarily believe in charity, but he believed that it was the duty of every fortunate individual to improve the opportunities afforded the less fortunate by allowing them to help themselves. He was thus a strong advocate in offering remedial relief and comfort to the sick and helpless. Monroe Anderson was indeed a rare individual whose values, along with those shared by his partners, led to the remarkable success of Anderson, Clayton & Company.[31]

Aside from strategic action, Anderson, Clayton's growth and expansion may also be credited to the direction and management style of its founders, including that of Monroe Anderson. On one occasion, Anderson told his friend and lawyer, Col. William B. Bates, that his success was due to his belief in the basic principle that "it was axiomatic that neither an individual nor people as a whole can ever be happy or prosper without hard work, thrift, and self-denial; that laziness and profligate spending inevitably lead to misery, poverty, and sorrow." His personal habits exemplified this conviction. Described by his family as quiet and soft-spoken, Monroe never smoked, drank, or used profane language. He was a very principled man who believed in hard work, self-denial, and exceptional frugality.[32]

Having a sense of humor and hobbies for relaxation were necessary antidotes to the long hours cotton merchants had to work. This was a year-round dilemma and not just a characteristic of the busy buying season. Anderson consistently worked from early in the morning until very late at night. While some cotton offices closed at noon on Saturdays, the employees of Anderson, Clayton & Company rarely indulged in such practices. As the lone resident manager of the firm in Houston, Monroe frequently used Saturday as a meeting day or a day to complete

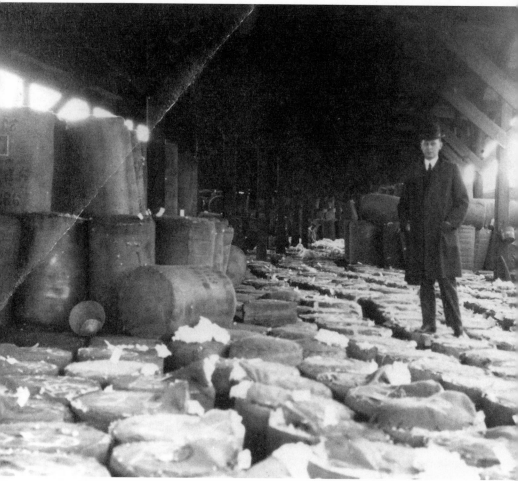

*Monroe D. Anderson standing on bales of cotton. RG-E-61-5, Houston Metropolitan Research Center, Houston Public Library.*

administrative duties. Aside from long days, Anderson cultivated an image of himself as a miser or scrooge when it came to money. It was his job to monitor the company's finances and expenditures. Since the company relied upon a tremendous amount of bank credit, he was known for always searching for a new way to save a dime. Perhaps for this reason and because of the growth of the company, in 1915 Anderson moved again, away from the stately Austin Street neighborhood to the Bender Hotel. Frank V. Bender and his brother, E. L., had opened the ten-story hotel in

1912. The building was striking in appearance, closer to the Anderson, Clayton offices in the Cotton Exchange Building, and offered rooms for a very good value, a perfect arrangement for Anderson.[33]

As Anderson, Clayton continued to grow, the need for more efficient and diversified transportation to move cotton increased. Ben Clayton's considerable past experience in shipping methods meant that he was as knowledgeable about the steamship industry as he was about railroads. As the Port of Houston neared completion in 1914, the opportunity that it provided for the firm could not be ignored. Monroe Anderson had successfully cultivated new financial relations with major banks, and now the company's other pressing need, better access to transportation, could be addressed.

At first, the partners thought it might be better to set up an office in Galveston. Ben Clayton and the others visited the island to assess the viability of such a move. Thomas Anderson remembered the family stories in which his father, Frank, after one exploratory trip, commented that "pirates had settled the island, and their descendants were still in control." In another account, after moving to Houston in May 1915, Ben Clayton went down to Galveston in mid-August with his wife, Julia, where they unwittingly encountered the 1915 hurricane. The rain and the wind were relentless, and Ben's car did not have windshield wipers. On the drive back to Houston, Ben was able to see only about ten feet in front of him while the water rose up over the running board of the car. Julia allegedly turned to Ben and sweetly said, "Ben Clayton, you may move your cotton company to Galveston, but I will never live there." After these events, Galveston was no longer a consideration. Instead, later that year, Ben Clayton began to establish the transportation and trading operations for the firm in Houston. The following year, Will Clayton moved his family to Houston, so that now both of the Clayton brothers had set up their families in homes in the best residential area of the city. By the time the Claytons moved to Houston, Anderson, Clayton had grown to a book value of $1 million. Monroe, always concerned about efficiency, continued to live in the Main-Bender Hotel close to the office. By contrast, Frank Anderson never moved to Houston, choosing instead to oversee the firm's business activities in Oklahoma City, where he continued to manage the grading, buying, and selling of cotton in that area.[34]

While Houston's economic growth matched its increase in population, its cultural venues were developing as well. The Houston Symphony Orchestra was founded in 1913; the Houston Art League received a significant donation from J. S. Cullinan in 1916 for a piece of land that would become the Museum of Fine Arts, which eventually opened in 1924. By 1915, Houston had 190 miles of paved streets and fifteen miles of electric streetcar lines. The city was clearly on its way to becoming a major economic stronghold in the South, and Anderson, Clayton & Company was carving out an ever-expanding niche in this growing market. Ultimately, the decision to move the company's headquarters to Houston facilitated the firm's handling of substantially larger amounts of product, since transporting huge volumes of cotton was no longer an issue. Houston, with its growing list of amenities and geographical location, was perfect in so many ways. Anderson, Clayton & Company was now positioned in a major railroad center, had easy access to a deepwater port, enjoyed relationships with a growing and abundantly stable banking industry, and was situated in one of the top cotton-producing states in the country.[35]

By 1916, Anderson, Clayton had established its headquarters in Houston, opened branch offices in New Orleans and Savannah, built its first major cotton warehouse in Houston, and opened a foreign office in Le Havre, France. Europe was engulfed by World War I at this time, however, which would change the fortunes of all cotton companies in the United States and would especially prove to be a turning point for Anderson, Clayton. Before the conflict, European firms held the upper hand and bought cotton grown in America on "CIF Terms." In other words, European firms paid for the cost, insurance, and freight to move cotton from US ports to the main European destinations of Bremen, Liverpool, and Le Havre. As the war continued, though, it became apparent that European firms would not be able to provide these measures, making it necessary to store cotton in the United States where it was grown. Anderson, Clayton & Company quickly seized upon this opportunity by building warehouses at the new Port of Houston, culminating in 1923 with the construction of the Long Reach warehouse and docks. Long Reach was the largest private warehouse and shipping facility located at the Turning Basin of the Houston Ship Channel. The warehouse contained several cotton compresses, and the docks were large enough to accommodate eight freighters at one time. Ultimately, World War I had proved the catalyst for major change within the global cotton industry. Anderson, Clayton & Company quickly took advantage of the opportunity, and now Europe was no longer the dominant player in the world of cotton. Indeed, the demand for cotton both during and after the war spurred the company on to expand its foreign office operations into new countries, including England, Germany, Italy, Japan, and China.[36]

By the early 1920s, the significant growth of the company resulted in two important changes. First, the partners decided to charter their business as a Texas joint stock association. This meant that should a partner withdraw from the firm or die, he or his estate had to sell, and the remaining partners would be forced to buy his interest at book value. Second, after the completion of the new Houston Cotton Exchange building in 1924, Anderson, Clayton & Company moved in, setting up offices on the entire eleventh floor and on part of the tenth floor as well. Monroe's office in the northwest corner of the eleventh floor provided a spectacular view of downtown. Meanwhile, Frank Anderson remained in Oklahoma City, where he had become known as a prominent community leader and a "quiet philanthropist." He served as president of the Oklahoma State Cotton Exchange, director of two banks, and president of several cotton-related firms. His son, Thomas Anderson, recalled that the Anderson, Clayton office in Oklahoma City was located on Harvey Street near the Rock Island Railroad, on "the upper floor of a [building that housed] the publisher of a farm and ranch newspaper. The office had few amenities and was reached by iron stairs, more industrial than commercial, with a good view of the noisy, spinning presses through a glass wall." Sometime during the early 1920s, when the Cotton Exchange in Oklahoma City constructed a new twelve-story building, Anderson, Clayton leased the eleventh floor just below the cotton trading room. The Oklahoma office, then, was still a significantly profitable asset to the company, and a few of Frank's sons had already joined their father to work for the firm.[37]

In 1924, shortly before Christmas, tragedy struck when Frank suffered an attack of appendicitis. His appendix burst, and Burdine rushed him to the hospital. Unfortunately, without antibiotics, the onset of peritonitis was likely. Frank fought the illness for three days while his wife remained at his side, but finally succumbed on December 15, 1924.

Burdine was devastated by his death, and although the funeral was held in the parlor of the family's home, she was unable to come downstairs to attend. His partners at Anderson, Clayton, true to their agreement, paid Frank's estate about $5 million, his share of the company based on the firm's book value at the time of his death. Frank left his family well off, and his will stated that his brother, Monroe, would be the trustee for the three youngest sons' portion of the estate. At the age of twenty-five, they would be on their own, but the years between their father's death and that time proved to be a financially profitable time for their estates. With Monroe's ability to manage money, he not only increased the value of their estates, but two of them were rewarded with more than double the value.[38]

By 1925, twenty-one years after founding the firm, only three original partners remained. Burdine Anderson stayed in Oklahoma until 1928, when her son, Thomas, finished high school. At that point, she moved to Houston and had a Mediterranean-style home built on South Boulevard to be close to the people she loved. Monroe came by almost daily, especially on Sundays, for dinner. Burdine was known for keeping fresh bouquets of flowers, and Monroe "borrowed" many a bouquet as he left on his way to visit a lady friend. Although Anderson enjoyed the company of women, primarily "beautiful widows," he remained a bachelor his entire life. According to Anderson family lore, a young Monroe had proposed to a sweetheart while he lived in Jackson, but she rejected his proposal, something from which he apparently never recovered.[39]

But by the mid-1920s, this unassuming bachelor was part of a firm that, like so many other US businesses, "roared" to prosperity during the so-called Roaring Twenties. Anderson, Clayton & Company, the cotton-trading firm established by two sets of brothers in rural Oklahoma in 1904, had become a successful global firm headquartered in Houston. The business-friendly city had all of the resources the company required for success, including stable banks, abundant railroad transportation, a deepwater seaport, and many developing cultural amenities. But public health in the city remained problematic, something that certainly had not gone unnoticed by Monroe Anderson.

Ultimately, as Anderson, Clayton & Company continued to establish its presence in Houston, the firm needed to engage the services of attorneys to handle its legal affairs. The ensuing success of Anderson, Clayton also contributed to the establishment and rise of a Houston law firm, Fulbright, Crooker, Freeman & Bates. Although alliances between corporate Houston and the city's lawyers were common, the relationship that developed between the principals of Fulbright, Crooker, Freeman & Bates and their clients at Anderson, Clayton & Company would have an enduring impact on Houstonians for generations to come.

# Chapter 3

## *The Legal Team*

### Fulbright, Crooker, Freeman & Bates

While the city of Houston provided the setting in which the cotton firm Anderson, Clayton & Company achieved global prominence and earned Monroe D. Anderson a sizable fortune, the law firm known for most of its history as Fulbright & Jaworski LLP played a key role as the company's legal advisor. In time, these attorneys also had a central, contributing part in both creating Monroe Anderson's foundation in 1936 and also serving as its primary trustees ever since. The law firm, established originally as Fulbright and Crooker in 1919 by Rufus Clarence Fulbright and John H. Crooker, was known as Fulbright, Crooker, and Freeman by 1936. It specialized in transportation issues and had as one of its earliest major clients the expanding cotton concern of Anderson, Clayton & Company. In order to fully understand the integral part the firm had in creating the M. D. Anderson Foundation and, later, the Texas Medical Center, it is useful to look briefly at the lawyers who formed the original firm and those who later established the Anderson Foundation. Generally, they came from fairly humble backgrounds and grew to maturity in an environment of stark reality that demanded hard work, developed strong character, and shaped them as young men to become the community leaders of their adulthood.

Coincidentally, the Fulbright family had once resided in Jackson, Tennessee, also the home of Frank Anderson and his brother Monroe. But like many folks from "back east," in 1875 Rufus T. Fulbright and his wife, Bertie (Welborn) Fulbright, moved to Texas to seek a new and better life. They settled in the northeast Texas community of New

Boston in Bowie County, just west of Texarkana and south of the Red River. Here, six years later, on October 6, 1881, their son Rufus Clarence Fulbright was born. Clarence grew up roaming the forested hills of this rural Texas community, attended Baylor University in Waco, and graduated in 1902 with a bachelor's degree in philosophy. After teaching school for a short time, he returned to Baylor and earned a master's degree in philosophy and then in 1906 was accepted at the University of Chicago Law School.[1]

During the law school's summer break of 1908, Clarence Fulbright visited Houston looking for employment opportunities in anticipation of his graduation the following year. The visit proved fruitful in that a firm where one of his Baylor classmates was employed, Andrews, Ball, and Streetman, offered him a job. During this visit he also became acquainted with John H. Freeman, who at the time worked at Stewart Abstract & Title Company. The two hit it off as friends, and when Freeman expressed his interest in the legal profession, Fulbright convinced him that he ought to attend the University of Chicago Law School. Freeman enrolled for classes that fall as Fulbright began his final year. Following his graduation in 1909, Clarence Fulbright returned to Houston to begin working at Andrews, Ball, and Streetman, where he took advantage of the firm's extensive railroad clientele—the firm had been representing railroads since 1902—to learn all he could about the railroad business. Fulbright quickly developed an expertise in commerce and rail shipping. This knowledge would serve him well during the 1920s and 1930s as railroads continued to thrive but were subjected to increased regulation from the Interstate Commerce Commission.[2]

In 1916 Fulbright's career began to take a new turn when the cotton firm Anderson, Clayton & Company moved its headquarters to Houston. World War I had begun two years earlier, and the US cotton industry was suffering as the strain on European nations increased. Because European customers could no longer afford to finance the purchase and storage of cotton from the United States, US firms had to change the way they conducted business. Anderson, Clayton saw this as an opportunity to expand its business, but the firm needed access to oceangoing transportation and warehouse space in which to store cotton. They chose Houston over Galveston as the best place to relocate their business and construct warehouses to store cotton until it was

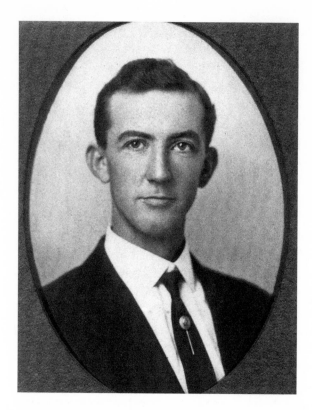

*R. C. Fulbright, ca. 1919. Courtesy of Fulbright & Jaworski LLP.*

needed by textile mills. Houston was already known as a railroad center, and the ease with which cotton could be shipped from growers around the country appealed to the firm. But, with each passing year, fluctuating railroad rates became an area of growing concern.

As mentioned earlier, Monroe D. Anderson had opened a small office for the cotton firm on the second floor of the old Cotton Exchange Building on Travis Street. Through his bankers at the Union National Bank, Anderson learned about the Andrews law firm and became acquainted with Clarence Fulbright. The fact that Fulbright's family originally was from Jackson, Tennessee, Monroe's hometown, likely helped to establish a rapport between the two men. In 1918 Anderson asked Fulbright to help the Anderson, Clayton firm in its dealings with the railroads and become the firm's rate counsel. But Clarence Fulbright could not represent both the cotton company and the railroad, because this would put him on both sides in rate issues, a clear conflict of interest. Consequently, Fulbright left the Andrews firm to start his own practice and accepted Anderson's offer to represent Anderson, Clayton & Company.[3]

While Clarence Fulbright was taking his first steps in the legal profession in Houston, John H. Freeman, as a student at the University of Chicago Law School, worked several jobs to pay his way and support himself. He had grown up on the north side of Houston in what was then known as the Fifth Ward, just a few blocks away from his friend and future law partner, John H. Crooker. Freeman's father, James D. Freeman, was a carpenter by trade and worked his way through the ranks to become a foreman for the Southern Pacific Railroad. John Henry Freeman was born in San Antonio, Texas, on October 23, 1886. His mother, Rose (Phelps) Freeman, was a native of San Antonio and had returned to her hometown to be with family when her baby arrived. Mother and son returned to Houston within a few weeks and settled into the family's modest home on Hardy Road. John Freeman attended Houston's public schools and graduated from Central High School. Years later, Freeman recalled during an interview that he worked "about five years" for an abstract company after graduating from high school in order to save up enough money to attend college. "I don't remember when I ever had any other idea [than to become a lawyer]," said Freeman. "There were no lawyers in my family immediately. And yet, that was my expectation always—to be a lawyer."[4]

Following the advice of his new friend, Clarence Fulbright, John Freeman enrolled at the University of Chicago Law School in the fall of 1908 and attended classes continuously until the end of the winter quarter in 1910. He had worked in the shoe department at Marshall Field's department store and at a campus bank to make ends meet, but in the end, the expenses and tuition were too great. Freeman was unable to complete his law degree. He later acknowledged that he "owed some money at that time" and returned to Houston, where he took a job with Houston Title Company to get his finances straight. Freeman noted that since he had received his legal training in Illinois, he "had to bone up on my Texas Law" to pass the bar examination before he could practice in his home state. He received his law license in 1913 but did not start to practice law until 1914 or 1915. In 1916 Freeman joined the law firm of former Houston mayor Ben Campbell and his associates,

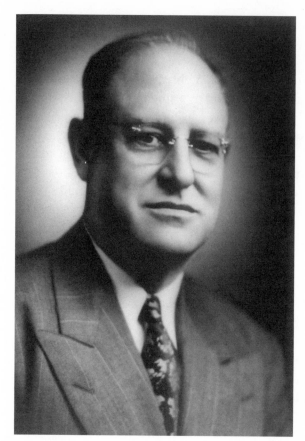

*John H. Freeman. Courtesy of Fulbright & Jaworski LLP.*

Sterling and Cyril Meyer, which then became known as Campbell, Meyer, Meyer, and Freeman. After the United States entered World War I, he took a leave of absence and in 1918 enlisted in the army. The war ended while Freeman was still stationed at Kelly Field in San Antonio. After he was discharged in 1919, he returned to work at what was then known as the firm of Campbell, Meyer, and Freeman. Freeman's years of work for abstract companies provided broad experience that enabled him to become very capable in real estate. His client list quickly grew and soon also included the State National Bank, originally established by John A. Wilkins and his brother, Horace M., as the State Bank and Trust Company in 1915.[5]

While John Freeman was studying law and preparing to take the Texas bar exam, his boyhood friend, John H. Crooker, was busy developing legal credentials of his own and making a reputation in Houston's legal community. John Crooker was born in Mobile, Alabama, on July 15, 1884, to Norman W. Crooker, a sailor, and his wife, Margaret (Kelton) Crooker. Norman Crooker died just two years later, ultimately causing his widow to migrate to Houston in 1893 in search of a better life for her family. They settled in the Fifth Ward, where nine-year-old Johnny Crooker began attending school. At age fourteen, with a seventh-grade education, he dropped out of school to help support his struggling family. Crooker worked a series of jobs and, more often than not, two jobs at a time. At the Southern Pacific Railroad, he worked in the tin shop, became an iron molder, and eventually served as a rail yard switchman. The hardworking young man also developed into a budding entrepreneur and engaged in several endeavors that included promoting excursion trains to the beach, operating a laundry wagon, and selling a variety of products from tea to educational materials for a correspondence school.[6]

During his rare moments of free time, Crooker began reading some of the correspondence school's books and developed a serious interest in the law and politics. He worked as a volunteer in an election campaign for constable in the city's Third Ward, and when his candidate won, the newly elected constable gratefully chose Crooker to serve as deputy constable. Months later, the twenty-three-year-old Crooker secured an appointment as clerk in the court of a justice of the peace, M. McDonald. This gave Crooker an opportunity to observe the legal system in action, which increased his interest and provided rudimentary experience. He began studying on his own with the encouragement of his wife and the assistance of his mother-in-law, Hortense Ward, who was also a lawyer, and with helpful tutoring from other attorneys with whom he had become acquainted. Although he did not attend a formal law school, in 1911 he passed the bar and acquired his law license. Within months, Justice of the Peace McDonald resigned, and the Harris County Commissioners Court appointed Crooker to serve out his term. In 1912 Crooker jumped headlong into politics and won election to his own full two-year term as justice of the peace.[7]

Both the law and politics perfectly suited John Crooker, and in 1914 he decided to challenge the incumbent, Richard Maury, for his seat as Harris County's district attorney. Maury died as a result of an automobile accident soon after Crooker entered the race, and the governor appointed attorney Clarence Kendall to serve the remainder of Maury's term. Crooker resigned his post as justice of the peace to devote all of his time to what became a very tough campaign. In a close finish, Crooker edged Kendall by just 116 votes to become the new district attorney. He soon developed a reputation as a fierce and vigorous prosecutor, quickly clearing a backlog of some 700 felony and murder cases and winning all but one of the jury cases. This "law and order" record led to Crooker's reelection in 1916.[8]

When the United States entered World War I, Crooker chose to enlist in the army, but before he left he played a role in three high-profile cases. In 1917 Houston was on the list to receive a military post, but the federal government threatened to cancel the creation of Camp Logan when officials became aware that just to the west of town the city had a thriving, legal, ten-block red-light district, known locally as the "Reservation." Among the owners were a number of prominent citizens whose identities remained secret. It was estimated that approximately 453 prostitutes resided in the area, under the watchful eyes of a few successful madams. During the late nineteenth and early twentieth centuries, prostitution flourished in Texas, as it did in many other states. Historian David Humphries wrote: "Many Texas communities routinely passed ordinances outlawing prostitution during the nineteenth century but paid only sporadic attention to them, influenced as their leaders were by the conventional wisdom that prostitution was ineradicable and therefore might as well be controlled. Community officials also had a keen appreciation of the hefty fines and rents prostitutes paid and the legions of male consumers they lured to town." The larger cities in Texas all had vice districts, and some, including Houston and Dallas, had legal vice zones or "reservations." The madams operated their establishments under the guise of "control" and in general enjoyed the support of many business and political leaders, some police, and also the "liquor and vice interests" that supported the districts. But in 1917 Secretary of War Newton D. Baker demanded that US soldiers in training camps across the country be protected from prostitution and venereal disease. Baker stated that cities that wanted to maintain or acquire military camps had to close down their vice districts and enforce antiprostitution ordinances, or they would lose the opportunity to have military encampments. Congress passed the National Selective Service Act of 1917, which had a provision that required a five-mile zone around military installations where saloons and prostitution were banned.[9]

A Texas law passed in 1907 legalized prostitution in the state, and in the following year a Houston city ordinance did the same within city limits. Houston's red-light district was so successful that by early 1917 the madams "enlisted" some 1,000 additional ladies who lived outside the Reservation in a futile attempt to keep up with the demand. City government seemed reluctant to close down the vice district, but when it appeared that Houston would miss out on the economic gain of hosting an army camp, a group including many of the city's business leaders and civic reformers formed the "Committee of One Hundred" to encourage the district attorney to close down the infamous houses of prostitution. With the state law and city ordinance still on the books, district attorney John Crooker did not know if he could win a conviction in these cases. Crooker essentially bluffed the sixty-four madams into going out of business by informing them that they had thirty days to close or they would face criminal prosecution. Being unaware of Crooker's doubts, by June 15, 1917, they had shuttered their businesses, and Houston became home to Camp Logan. Between March and August 1917, El Paso, Fort Worth, Galveston, San Antonio, and Waco also closed down their vice districts in an attempt to eliminate prostitution and comply with the War Department's mandate.[10]

Just weeks later, on August 23, 1917, black soldiers stationed at the newly opened Camp Logan reacted to weeks of racial abuse and Jim Crow segregation laws. The camp was to be the training base for the Illinois National Guard, and the army sent the Third Battalion of the black Twenty-fourth US Infantry, along with seven white officers, from Columbus, New Mexico, to Houston, where they were to guard the camp while it was under construction. But after repeated incidents of racial abuse, approximately 100 angry black soldiers marched on the city. In the rioting that followed, eleven white civilians, four white police officers, and four black soldiers were killed. In the aftermath of the riot, the Third Battalion was sent back to New Mexico. Later the army held three courts-martial at Fort Sam Houston in San Antonio, where, between November 1, 1917, and March 26, 1918, the military indicted 118 enlisted men of I Company for their part in the mutiny and riot. Although the trials were conducted outside of Harris County, the military invited Crooker to participate in the initial prosecution. Of the 110 soldiers who were convicted, 19 were hanged, and 63 were sentenced to life in prison. One of the soldiers was found incompetent to stand trial.[11]

Following his role in the Camp Logan court-martial, thirty-four-year-old John Crooker prepared to resign as district attorney to enlist in the army. But before leaving, he filed a suit to remove the executors of the George Hermann Estate. Hermann, a wealthy bachelor, had died in 1914 and left a large estate of $2.6 million, including land and $100,000, designated to construct a public charity hospital to serve the poor and infirm of Houston. Hermann had named T. J. Ewing Jr., J. J. Settegast, and John S. Steward as executors of his estate. After the will was settled in probate court, the three executors were to add four trustees to join them on a board that was to build and maintain a public charity hospital. But by 1917 the original executors of Hermann's will had not named the additional trustees and, in the eyes of many in the community, had failed to fulfill their responsibilities and possibly misused estate funds. Crooker filed suit, and soon after, Houston's mayor, A. Earl Amerman, also filed suit. Crooker then joined the army and left the lawsuit in the hands of James A. Elkins, the interim district attorney. Elkins soon brokered a settlement in which the court approved new trustees G. A. A. Brandt, William A. Childress, Henry F. MacGregor, and Ross Sterling. The original executors resigned and were replaced by T. P. Lee, Joseph F. Meyer, and Paul B. Timpson. But it would be another eight years before George Hermann's last wish was fulfilled and Hermann Hospital finally opened.[12]

Ironically, Crooker trained for a short time at Camp Logan and then received a transfer to Camp Kearney in La Jolla, California. He was promoted to major and was assigned as judge advocate of a division that was preparing to go overseas. When the Armistice was declared in November 1918, the army canceled the division's orders and sent Crooker to the Judge Advocate General's office in Washington, DC, where he finished his tour of duty and was discharged in August 1919.[13]

The man who became the fourth named partner in Fulbright, Crooker, Freeman & Bates, William Bartholomew Bates, was born on August 16, 1889, in the small East Texas community of Nat, about

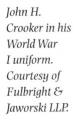

*John H.
Crooker in his
World War
I uniform.
Courtesy of
Fulbright &
Jaworski LLP.*

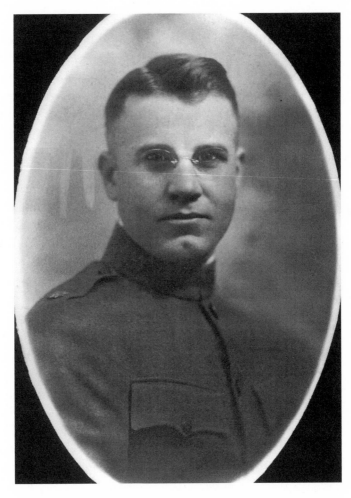

fourteen miles from Nacogdoches. He was the sixth of thirteen children of James Madison and Mary Frances (Cook) Bates. At the time of Bates's birth, the little community was known as Crossroads because of the Crossroads Cumberland Presbyterian Church. It was renamed Nat in 1895 in honor of local store owner Nathan (Nat) Jarrell, who became the first postmaster.[14]

Bates grew up on his family's farm in rural East Texas. His father grew cotton, and the family lived off the land, growing their own vegetables, raising chickens, and tending to a dairy cow. Like most boys growing up in the Texas countryside, Bates loved the outdoors, where he spent many happy days hunting raccoons, squirrels, and rabbits. His mother made most of the clothes for her large brood, which also included an abandoned boy whom the Bates family took in and raised as their own. "We raised cotton, corn, peanuts, sugar cane, and sweet potatoes," Bates recalled in 1973. "We always made three or four hundred gallons of syrup. We didn't use it all ourselves, but it was just like legal tender. You could get a day's work for a gallon of syrup or a bushel of corn. We didn't have much money, neither did anybody else. Most everything was barter."[15]

Bates attended the rural schools in the community and in 1911 earned an elementary school teaching certificate at Sam Houston State Teachers College in Huntsville, Texas. He taught for a year, and then both he and his brother, Jesse, enrolled in the University of Texas Law School. Although the assistant dean thought Bates was ill prepared for success in law school, he nevertheless graduated at the top of his class in 1915.[16]

After graduation, Bates found employment in Bay City with a lawyer, William Cash, who also owned an abstract company. During an interview years later, Bates recalled that he had arrived by train in Bay City, which is located about eighteen miles from the Gulf of Mexico, just hours before the hurricane of 1915. By midnight, as the full force of the storm slammed the community, Bates took shelter in a local hotel and later recalled that he could "hear the Gulf roaring at the time." The storm, which was considered to be worse than the 1900 storm that destroyed Galveston, blew out all the plate glass windows around the town's square.[17]

Bates worked in Bay City for about the next eighteen months, during which time he also organized a local Boy Scout troop. When the United States formally entered World War I on April 6, 1917, Bates, like many fellow Texans, enlisted in the armed forces. On May 12, 1917, he reported for officer training at Camp Leon Springs, near San Antonio, with a group of men consisting mainly of graduates from Texas A&M and the University of Texas. After what he described as "severe training . . . a heavy, rushed course," his group graduated on August 15 and reported to Camp Travis at Fort Sam Houston, where newly commissioned 2nd Lt. William B. Bates was assigned to Company E, 358th Infantry Regiment, 90th Division—the Texas/Oklahoma division. Many of the early arrivals in the division were sent overseas immediately to replace casualties, so it took several more months for the 90th to reach full strength. In June 1918 they shipped out by train to Long Island, New York, and then spent thirteen days at sea, en route to Liverpool, England, where they arrived on July 1. "The Fourth of July came along and our regiment was selected to celebrate in Liverpool," said Bates. "So, we marched down to the flat at the water's edge, right in front of an enormous statue of King George III. And that is where we held our program for the Fourth of July, 1918. The mayor [of Liverpool] gave us a big banquet that day. We enjoyed it because of the irony of the situation." Several days later they landed at Le Havre in France, where they endured more training, even as the sounds of cannon fire from the Battle of Château-Thierry provided background and what Bates described as "my first introduction to the war."[18]

*William B. Bates in his World War I uniform. Courtesy of Fulbright & Jaworski LLP.*

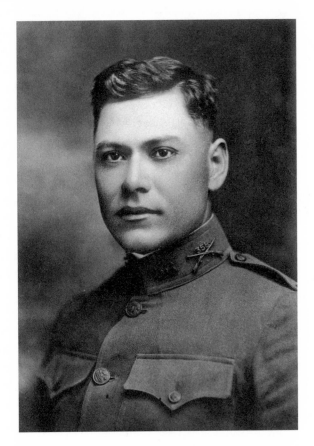

The 90th soon received orders to relieve the 1st Division on the front lines at Saint-Mihiel, the first major US offensive of the war. The US Army deployed along the southern edge of the Saint-Mihiel salient, which had been held by the Germans since 1914. By September of 1918, the Germans were in retreat when, on the morning of September 12, US troops under the command of Gen. John J. Pershing attacked. Caught by surprise, the Germans collapsed. Within thirty-six hours the Americans killed or wounded 5,000 Germans and captured over 13,000 prisoners and 466 guns while suffering 7,000 casualties.[19]

As Bates later recalled, "We had a very difficult time and lost about . . . 5,000 troops from our division. That [was] one of the largest losses of any individual [division] in the fight." During the fierce fighting, several officers were severely wounded, including Bates's company commander. Bates suffered a shrapnel wound in his arm, but because many officers had been killed or wounded, he remained in the fight. His company soon came under fierce fire from an enemy machine gun nest and was unable to dig in. Their new commander, Capt. Simpson, sent Bates, along with another officer and several men, to destroy these machine guns. French artillery had bombarded the area to destroy the barbed-wire entanglements laid out by the German troops, but as Bates and his men advanced, they discovered that much of the wire remained intact, forcing them to cut it and crawl through to go forward. "Just as we were emerging from the barbed wire," Bates recalled years later, "the enemy opened up on us. I dived into a shell hole and stayed there for two or three hours. I had to hug the ground as close as possible, keep my head down—the pack on my back was shot to pieces but they didn't get me. We lost seven men, including the other officer and our first sergeant, who were over on my left in the trench. They failed to keep their heads down, and both of them were killed. Another group finally came up on our left and got that machine gun nest." Bates received a citation for gallantry in action and was promoted to first lieutenant. He was wounded again during the last phase of the Meuse-Argonne campaign and received another citation for gallantry and promotion to captain. After the Armistice, the 90th Division served as part of the Army of Occupation. The division returned home, landing at Boston on July 6, 1919, and then was discharged at Camp Travis, near San Antonio, on July 16, 1919.[20]

Interestingly, his later title of colonel had nothing to do with his military service in World War I, but rather was an honorary title bestowed by Bates's friend and former classmate, Daniel J. Moody following Moody's election as governor of Texas in 1926. "I made speeches for him, and he was elected governor," said Bates. "He appointed me colonel on his staff. From that time on I have been Colonel Bates."[21]

He returned to Nacogdoches, where he and his brother wasted no time in opening a law firm, Bates and Bates, on August 1, 1919. During this time, Bates also decided to run for district attorney in the Second Judicial District of Texas, which at the time included Nacogdoches, Cherokee, and Angelina Counties. He won election in 1920, based in part on his war record. Prohibition was the law of the land at that time, and the Ku Klux Klan was strong in East Texas, too. Bates prosecuted violators of the prohibition laws and stood firmly against the Klan—a noble effort, but one that was not politically popular. When he ran for reelection in 1922, as he said later, "I had sent to the penitentiary for bootlegging a relative of almost everybody in the community. The Ku Klux Klan was popular in those counties, too. So, I was defeated by about 125 votes in each county." All along, Bates had planned eventually to practice civil law in either Houston or Dallas, but his electoral defeat moved that timetable forward considerably.[22]

During the time that Bates was preparing to run for district attorney and tame Texas' Second Judicial District, Clarence Fulbright and John Crooker began talking about forming a law firm together. Fulbright had opened a solo practice at the behest of Monroe D. Anderson in 1918 and handled all of the cotton firm's railroad rate matters. Crooker, who had returned to Houston from military service in August 1919, was looking for a new start in his legal career. Fulbright believed that Crooker, an experienced litigator and former district attorney, would bring a different skill set that would enhance his growing practice. During their conversations in the late summer of 1919, the two saw that the differences in their education and career paths, in fact, complemented each other. With a major client—Anderson, Clayton—already in the fold, on October 1, 1919, R. C. Fulbright and John H. Crooker announced that they had formed a "general civil practice of the law under the firm name of Fulbright & Crooker" with offices in the Union National Bank Building.[23]

Throughout the 1920s and 1930s, both the Anderson, Clayton and the Fulbright & Crooker firms continued to grow. The years of the Great Depression affected Houston, but not as severely as other parts of the country. The demand for cotton remained strong, and railroads continued to provide a major form of shipping and general cross-country transportation. One of the results of this was that Fulbright & Crooker was handling a large portion of Anderson, Clayton's legal affairs. By the end of 1922, William B. Bates was looking for a new job, having just been defeated in his bid for reelection as district attorney. During his brief foray into county politics, he had gained much practical courtroom experience. His term as district attorney officially ended on December 31, 1922, and he immediately began looking for a new employment opportunity. Bates came to Houston to interview for a position as trial lawyer with Vinson & Elkins on Saturday, December 22, 1922. While he waited to hear whether he would be hired, Bates went out for a walk down Main Street and happened to see a former classmate from the University of Texas, Sam Polk, who was working for Fulbright & Crooker. Polk was happy to see his old friend and suggested that he go with him, right then, to the Fulbright offices. As Bates recalled years later, "The office was still open, and Mr. Crooker had gone home, but Mr. Fulbright was still there." His friend told Fulbright all about Bates, his school years, military service, and term as district attorney. "He was a good man to have for your friend," said Bates. Fulbright acknowledged that the firm was growing fast and that they could probably use another attorney in the coming months. He told Bates that he would like his partner to meet him. Bates arranged to return to meet John Crooker on the next Wednesday, the day after Christmas.[24]

Bates's colleagues in Nacogdoches sent letters of recommendation on his behalf to Fulbright & Crooker. Following the interview on December 26, Crooker and Fulbright took Bates to lunch at the Houston Club, where they discussed his salary and offered him a position with the firm. The $200 per month was much less than the $350 he had earned as district attorney, but Bates was excited about the opportunity. "So, January 1, 1923, just as the horns were blowing and the bells were ringing the old year out and the New Year in, I took the train at Nacogdoches," said Bates. "I arrived in Houston about 7:00 or 8:00 that morning and went to the office of Fulbright & Crooker. In those days and for many years thereafter, the firm worked every New Year's Day . . . felt like they had to start the year off right."[25]

Bates stated that he was hired by the firm primarily to assist Crooker in the district court. His first case involved a suit that Anderson, Clayton had filed against a merchant in Vernon, Texas, over an excessive $5,000 payment for a shipment of cotton. Although Bates faced Joseph Weldon Bailey, reputed to be one of the country's outstanding constitutional lawyers, he kept his poise and scored a victory when Bailey's attempt to move the trial out of Houston by using a plea of privilege was denied. Bates and Bailey then settled the suit out of court.[26]

When Bates joined Fulbright and Crooker, the firm had been in existence for barely three years, but it was already well known and highly regarded for being so young. The firm's principal client at this time was Anderson, Clayton & Company. The Port of Houston was in its early stages of development, and both railroad and water freight rates were important to the cotton firm as well as to the port. The income tax was a relatively new development, and tax litigation was just beginning as well. By this time, Clarence Fulbright was recognized as one of Houston's eminent lawyers in both freight rates and tax litigation. John Crooker, who had recently returned from the army, had earned a distinguished record of service in the judge advocate's department. He had been district attorney in Houston before entering the army and had been recognized as one of the most able men ever to hold that office. Crooker also had the reputation of being one of the best trial lawyers at the Houston Bar.[27]

John Freeman joined Fulbright and Crooker one year after Bates, on January 1, 1924. "He had been a partner in the firm of Campbell, Myer, and Freeman for several years and was well established as an able and successful lawyer," said Bates. "He was a director and attorney for the State National Bank at the time, so our firm not only gained a great lawyer, it acquired its first bank representation. The name of the firm was changed to Fulbright, Crooker, & Freeman." Bates was not alone in his admiration for John Freeman. He was described as a "prodigious worker" whom colleagues compared to "a giant river, wide and deep and moving with great force" and a "steady and unobtrusive influence on the firm's development."[28]

During the next few years, Fulbright, Crooker, & Freeman provided legal services for Anderson, Clayton & Company as the cotton firm continued to grow. Anderson, Clayton soon had interests around the world, "wherever cotton was grown, bought, sold, or made into thread and cloth." It was, then, an internationally known business on the way to becoming the largest cotton firm in the world when the law firm assigned Colonel Bates to handle much of Anderson, Clayton's legal work.[29]

Years later, Bates recalled working with both Ben and Will Clayton and his first meeting with Monroe D. Anderson. "I guess I remember Ben Clayton first, because he's the one I worked with first," said Bates. Ben Clayton asked Bates to examine abstracts for 400 acres of land that Anderson, Clayton & Company had purchased for a textile mill. Bates was familiar with land work and in short order examined the land titles and returned all of the documents that Anderson, Clayton had provided. This attention to detail and protocol earned high praise from Ben Clayton. "He thought that was unusual for a young lawyer," said Bates. "He said I was the first lawyer they'd ever had who brought back everything without being asked for it."[30]

Bates's first work for Will Clayton came on a December Saturday in 1927. Clayton called Bates at his home and asked if he would accompany him to New York. "When?" asked Bates. "In about thirty minutes," replied Clayton. The two men spent the next ten days together in New York, and Bates was surprised that Clayton displayed such a high level of trust in the young attorney. "He seemed to have confidence in me and, naturally, that inspired my confidence," said Bates. They returned to Houston for Christmas, and then Clayton sent Bates to Greenville, South Carolina, on the same matter. Clayton entrusted Bates with the responsibility of organizing a new corporation to resolve a problem that involved some 800 bales of cotton and $1 million in forged warehouse receipts. The firm recognized Bates's contributions and on January 1, 1928, made William B. Bates a partner. Twelve years later, on June 1, 1940, Bates became a named partner when the firm changed its name to Fulbright, Crooker, Freeman & Bates. Perhaps the most important relationship to emerge out of the firm's work for Anderson, Clayton & Company was the friendship that developed over time between William B. Bates and Monroe D. Anderson. "The first time I remember meeting M. D. Anderson, he was in his office over the Houston Trunk Factory at Main and Rusk," said Bates. "Anderson, Clayton had their offices up there then. Mr. Anderson and I got along together very well. We fished together." Bates remembered his friend as someone who "lived simply and unostentatiously." Although Anderson had a "wide acquaintance," many thought him reticent and shy. "Only a few knew him intimately," said Bates. "Those who did greatly admired and loved him."[31]

All through the next decade, Fulbright, Crooker & Freeman provided most of the legal services for Anderson, Clayton & Company, which also helped to foster a level of trust and friendship among Freeman, Bates, and Anderson. By the mid-1930s, Anderson's health was in decline, and he turned to his trusted attorneys and friends, William Bates and John Freeman, to help him with his estate planning. The business and personal connections that they developed during these years created a comfortable setting in which they could talk freely and envision what Anderson could do with his vast fortune as he began to think about the inevitable. Ultimately, they formulated a plan to put Anderson's fortune into a charitable foundation that would have a lasting, positive impact far beyond what these men might have imagined. For more than seventy years, attorneys from the Fulbright firm have kept the faith with Monroe Anderson in their careful stewardship of his foundation. During the meetings and conversations that led to the creation of the M. D. Anderson Foundation, however, none of the principals involved in the discussions realized how little time remained in Anderson's life. Soon enough, Bates and Freeman would have to find a suitable means to ensure that their friend's wishes would be fulfilled and that his legacy would not be squandered—as had nearly happened to the George Hermann estate—and do so without much guidance from their friend. With the Depression dragging on and the world about to erupt in the conflagration of World War II, William B. Bates, John H. Freeman, and Monroe D. Anderson had much about which to be concerned as they began to formulate the plans for a foundation that ultimately would change the face of Houston and have a lasting impact on health care in the United States.

# Chapter 4

## *Legacy*

### Creating the M. D. Anderson Foundation

When Monroe Dunaway Anderson established his charitable foundation in 1936, few Houstonians other than his close friends, family, and the employees of Anderson, Clayton & Company knew much about him. But Anderson created a legacy almost unparalleled in Houston's history, a philanthropic foundation that in turn would benefit countless individuals, particularly in the areas of education, health care, and cancer research and treatment. It is ironic that a man who was rather shy and shunned the spotlight in life now is known far and wide due to the generous efforts of the M. D. Anderson Foundation and the top-ranked cancer research hospital that bears his name: the University of Texas M. D. Anderson Cancer Center in Houston.

By 1936 Monroe Anderson was one of the remaining founding partners of the global cotton firm Anderson, Clayton & Company. By the 1930s, the firm had grown from its humble origins as a small cotton-trading company based in Oklahoma City to a worldwide giant that had a net worth of some $100 million. Although the world was dealing with the effects of global recession and both Japan and Germany had threatened aggressive moves against their neighbors, Anderson, Clayton continued to prosper, making Monroe Anderson a very wealthy man in the process. By 1936, with obvious signs of declining health, Anderson turned to his trusted attorneys and close friends, William B. Bates and John H. Freeman of the law firm Fulbright, Crooker, & Freeman, to help him with his estate planning. Anderson was concerned that if he should die, his partners in Anderson, Clayton would not have enough financial resources to buy out his share of the firm without liquidating the company.

As discussed earlier, in 1904 brothers Frank and Monroe Anderson and William and Benjamin Clayton organized Anderson, Clayton & Company as a firm engaged in cotton merchandising, ginning, and other related products and activities. By 1920, Anderson, Clayton & Company had assets of some $7 million. On May 31, 1920, the partners converted the firm into a joint stock association and brought six employees into the business for small amounts of stock in the association. Both sets of brothers, the Andersons and the Claytons, as directors and principal shareholders in the association, agreed that any of them could request dissolution and that in the event one of the members should die, the association should purchase their interest "at the book value thereof as determined by the directors." This agreement, sadly, was put to the test when Frank E. Anderson died in December 1924. After going through probate and the legal process, the association purchased the stock held by Frank Anderson, 16,293 shares, for $5.7 million during the next fiscal year ending May 31, 1926.[1]

Less than three years later, in March 1929, Benjamin Clayton determined that because of his poor health at that time, he should take his leave from the business. Still feeling the effects on his health from his earlier bout with pneumonia and other illnesses, he decided to retire from the company in May 1929. Although only forty-seven years of age, he desired to cut back his work hours to only three a day and move to his cattle ranch in New Mexico. He held about one-third of the stock, worth approximately $12 million, and requested that he be able to cash in his shares. The firm consulted with investment bankers to raise the cash, either through the sale of preferred stock or debentures. But after the stock market crashed in October 1929, the company's stock could no longer be sold at a reasonable value. And because the cotton merchandising business was very cash dependent, the firm needed all of its working capital just to function in business. Will Clayton and Monroe Anderson were unwilling to sell corporate assets to pay off Ben Clayton's claim and feared that they might not have sufficient resources to keep the business going if any other principals withdrew from the association or died. In November 1929 they finally worked out a plan to organize a holding company, Anderson-Clayton Securities Corporation, to acquire all of the Anderson, Clayton association stock and pay off Ben Clayton in installments.[2]

During the next few years, Anderson, Clayton & Company dealt with its share of issues and concerns as the Great Depression lingered into the 1930s. Anecdotal evidence suggests that the experience of trying to buy out Ben Clayton's interests in the company, the pressure of trying to maintain a successful business during the Depression, and his growing disdain for Franklin Roosevelt's policies all weighed on Monroe Anderson. By 1936, as he struggled with failing health, including kidney disease and congestive heart failure, his net worth was somewhere in the range of $18–20 million. Being a lifelong bachelor with no children, Anderson determined that it was time for him to take the necessary steps to protect both the company and his own desires for dispersing his personal fortune in the event of his death. Years later, William B. Bates noted, "I was the attorney that took care of Anderson Clayton. Mr. Anderson almost had to establish a foundation, because it would have been difficult for the company to exist if he hadn't." Bates observed that by the mid-1930s, the three major remaining partners, William L. Clayton, Monroe D. Anderson, and Lamar Fleming, were all obligated in the event of the death of one of the partners to buy out the deceased's interest at book value. Bates recalled that "Mr. Anderson was getting up in years. His health wasn't the best [and] he was worried about the situation, if he should die soon, because Anderson, Clayton was becoming a big concern. With the tax laws then in effect, it would have been impossible for [major partners Will Clayton and Lamar Fleming] to have bought his interest without liquidating the company." In addition, Monroe Anderson was very fond of all the people in the firm, about 800 employees, and he knew many of them by name. He felt a sense of loyalty and responsibility to the employees and did not want anything to happen that might force the firm to close, causing the layoff of the workers in the midst of the Depression. Through the creation of a charitable foundation, his fortune could go into it without being taxed, and Anderson, Clayton & Company would not have to be liquidated.[3]

Monroe Anderson thus began a series of deep, earnest conversations with his lawyers about his estate and the options for creating a foundation. According to William Bates, Anderson had long been interested in medicine and public health. The three men, Anderson, Bates, and Freeman, began to explore how to create a vehicle for Anderson's wealth to have an impact for the betterment of mankind. "In fact, he came by my offices, [or] pulled me to his own office, every morning for two or three years [while] we were working on that," Bates recalled. On June 9, 1936, the three men met in Bates's office, and Anderson signed the papers establishing the M. D. Anderson Foundation. Anderson, Bates, and Freeman also served as the foundation's first board of trustees (see appendix 1). In addition to organizing the foundation, Bates and Freeman also helped Anderson prepare a will in which he named three of his nephews, James, Leland, and Thomas Anderson, as executors of his estate.[4]

Years later, Bates recalled of his friend, "He refused to be rushed on important matters, insisting on adequate time to think and meditate before reaching decisions of consequence." Bates stated that while Anderson did not believe in personal charity for the individual, with the exception of the disabled and afflicted, he did believe strongly in giving relief and comfort to the sick and helpless. He also believed in "improving the opportunity" for people to advance themselves.[5]

The trust indenture he signed in Bates's office that June day in 1936 spelled out the purpose of the new foundation.

> All of the net income, being all of the income after payment of taxes and expenses, shall be used and applied by the Trustees to some one or more of the charitable uses and purposes herein set forth, that is to say:
>
> To the improvement of working conditions among workers generally, as well as among particular classes of unskilled and agricultural workers;
>
> To the establishment, support, and maintenance of hospitals, homes, and institutions for the care of the sick, the young, the aged, the incompetent, and the helpless among the people;
>
> To the improvement of living conditions among people generally as well as in particular sections or localities;
>
> To the promotion of health, science, education, and advancement and diffusion of knowledge and understanding among people.[6]

Anderson made an initial contribution of $10,000 to launch the foundation. During the next three years he made several deposits that increased the corpus to about $300,000. According to Bates, the foundation's first grant, made during Anderson's lifetime, was "a token donation" of $150 to the Houston Junior League to help with the purchase of eyeglasses for needy schoolchildren. The trustees continued to make small donations to the Junior League program whenever asked, about $1,700 total, until the Junior League secured financing for the eyeglasses program from other donors.[7]

Having established his charitable foundation, Monroe Anderson continued to discuss plans for it with Bates, and often with Freeman too, nearly every day. Anderson's nephew, Thomas D. Anderson, recalled that by 1936 his uncle "Mon" was in pretty poor physical condition: "He fished a lot and hunted some [but] had very little interest in symphonies or operas, things of that sort. He took virtually no exercise." He enjoyed fishing with Bates and numbered among his small circle of friends Freeman and several banking colleagues, including Horace Wilkins, who later succeeded Anderson as trustee of his foundation, Clarence Malone, head of the Guardian Trust Company, and Robert A. Welch, a businessman and fellow bachelor who became wealthy from his oil, mineral, and real estate interests. Anderson preferred to remain out of the limelight. He quietly supported some local causes but was "a philanthropist who did not want to be identified as such," according to his nephew.[8]

Monroe Anderson frequently enjoyed lunch with business colleagues at the Majestic Grill, located in the same building that housed the Majestic Theater, on Travis Street at Rusk, two blocks from his home in the Texas State Hotel. For years, he had resided at the Bender Hotel, which also was located downtown, but in 1931 the hotel management informed the residents that the electricity would be turned off and the building closed for renovations. Anderson seemingly did not believe this was true. He came home one evening and found the lights out and the elevators no longer working. The bell captain, Oscar Collins, helped him pack and carry his belongings down six flights of stairs and move to the new Texas State Hotel, which recently had opened that same year on the corner of Fannin and Rusk.[9]

On October 7, 1938, Anderson met Arthur Fisher, a vice president

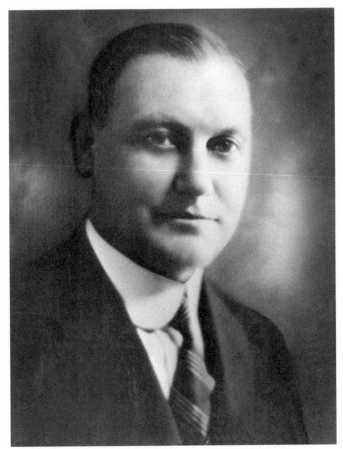

*Monroe D. Anderson in his later years. Courtesy of John P. McGovern Historical Collections and Research Center, Texas Medical Center Library.*

of the National Bank of Commerce (later Texas Commerce Bank), for lunch at the Majestic Grill. The two friends took their customary seats at the counter near the front of the diner. While they were eating their lunch, Anderson complained that his arm had become numb.[10] As he rubbed and thrashed his arm, attempting to restore feeling, Fisher spotted his friend's nephew, Thomas Anderson, who coincidentally was also enjoying a lunch at the Majestic. Years later, Thomas Anderson recalled that Arthur Fisher came to his table with a concerned look on his face and said, "Your uncle is having a problem. You had better come and see about him." Anderson rushed to aid his uncle. "He was thrashing his

[left] arm like it was going to sleep. His face was flushed; we knew he was in distress. I wasn't very old but I knew, I could tell when somebody had had a stroke."[11]

Anderson wanted to take his uncle directly to the hospital, but Monroe refused and insisted on returning to his room at the Texas State Hotel. "We immediately hailed a taxicab and transported him to the hotel's Fannin Street entrance," said Anderson. "We beckoned two bellmen and they seated him in a chair, picked him up chair and all, and carried him up to his room. We made him as comfortable as we could and called his physician, Dr. Joe Henry Graves, the younger brother of the renowned Dr. Marvin L. Graves." When Dr. Graves arrived, he found Monroe Anderson flushed and excited and gave him a sedative to calm him. They arranged for nurses to come to the hotel to attend to Monroe. That evening, Anderson's nephews Thomas, James, and Leland met with Dr. Graves in the hotel lobby. "He told us that our uncle had suffered for some time from Bright's disease, a kidney ailment that brings about inflammation of the kidneys. It can be quite painful and ultimately lead to serious consequences," said Thomas Anderson. "But, at the moment, the stroke gave him the greatest concern. He asked us to get our uncle to a hospital right away, the nearest one being the Baptist Memorial Hospital, then located downtown." Monroe finally agreed to go to the hospital, and his nephews called for a taxi to take him the short distance. With his side still sagging and numb, physicians immediately diagnosed the stroke and gave Anderson nitroglycerin. Since Dr. Graves did not have staff privileges at Baptist Memorial Hospital, Dr. James Greenwood Jr. took over care and attended Monroe Anderson for the remainder of his life.[12]

Anderson remained hospitalized and soon became weary of the daily hospital routine. Thomas Anderson recalled that despite being restless and bored, his uncle still retained at least some of his sense of humor. "I remember one occasion when Dr. Greenwood came into the room and, to test the patient's weakened hand to see if he could recognize a coin by touch, he placed a fifty-cent piece in that hand and told him to squeeze firmly. Uncle Mon squeezed all right, but he could not identify the coin from touch. He quickly took the coin with his good hand and slipped it into his pajama pocket, looking up at the doctor all the while in innocent anticipation of the next step in the examination.

We thought we saw in his eyes a hint of the playfulness all of us had known for so many years. He returned the coin the next morning saying, 'You forgot this.'" Although Monroe never regained use of his left side, he became determined that he would not spend his last days cooped up in the hospital. After six months of being hospitalized, he assigned his nephews the task of finding a house in which he could convalesce and arranged for one of his nurses, a Miss Avery, to organize a team of nurses who could provide home care for him.[13]

A realtor found a home on Sunset Boulevard near Rice University, and in late April or early May 1939 Monroe Anderson moved into the only home outside of a hotel that he had lived in since his childhood years in Jackson, Tennessee. The house was located on a tree-lined street and surrounded by beautifully manicured lawns, flowers, shrubs, and trees. "We hoped he would find inspiration and strength from his new home with its lovely surroundings and from his family and his friends, who so fervently wished him well," said Thomas Anderson. Dr. Greenwood continued to provide medical care, and Anderson tried to regain use of his left side, even attempting to walk with a cane. Nurse Avery, a very capable manager, and a small staff of nurses did their best to make him comfortable, but as Thomas Anderson recalled, his uncle's last days "were pretty miserable." Monroe never regained use of his left arm, and his leg did not function either. "I do not know whether he was in any particular pain, but he had essentially the life of an invalid from the time of his stroke until the time of his death." Anderson struggled with his combined illnesses, but at 7:40 on Sunday morning, August 6, 1939, he suffered a severe heart attack and died in his home at the age of sixty-six.[14]

As news of Anderson's death spread throughout Houston's banking and business communities, his friends, colleagues, and community leaders paid tribute. Will Clayton, who at the time was chairman of the board of Anderson, Clayton & Company, said, "It is a great sorrow to me to lose him. He was both my partner and my friend." The *Houston Post* editorialized that Anderson "was a builder with enterprise and vision." Later in the week, the Houston Cotton Exchange and Board of Trade's board of directors issued a resolution of sympathy and remembered Anderson as "one of the most valuable members of the exchange." Rev. T. E. Roberts of the First Presbyterian Church conducted Anderson's funeral service at noon on Tuesday, August 8. Among the many friends listed as pallbearers were such noteworthy Houstonians as Clarence Malone, William B. Bates, John Freeman, Holger Jeppesen, and Robert A. Welch. Grieving friends and family made the journey to Jackson, Tennessee, where Monroe Dunaway Anderson's remains were cremated and laid to rest in the family plot, near the graves of his parents.[15]

Following Anderson's death, on Thursday, August 10, 1939, Fulbright, Crooker, and Freeman and the executors of his estate, nephews Thomas, Leland, and James Anderson, filed the estate tax return and papers to process the will in probate court. In a statement attorneys for the law firm said, "The establishment and setting into operation of this foundation by Mr. Anderson represented for him the culmination of a lifetime of achievement and useful public effort." As word of the filing became known, Houston newspapers reported the rumors that Anderson had "left a considerable amount" to be paid into the M. D. Anderson Foundation, but few people actually knew how large an estate he had left. It was valued at approximately $20 million, of which $1 million was designated for his heirs and the remaining $19 million for his foundation. On Sunday, August 13, 1939, the *Houston Post* editorial page noted Anderson's generosity: "To an impressive list of Houston philanthropists who have given millions to make life better for their fellows is added the name of M. D. Anderson . . . . Thus, the M. D. Anderson Foundation takes its place as one of the major benefactions made available to the people of Houston and Texas by a Houstonian who returned to society much of the wealth he accumulated during a successful and useful career."[16]

With such a large portion of the estate going to the charitable foundation, beyond the reach of federal tax agents, it took some two years before the will was probated and the funds transferred to the foundation. During that time the executors managed the estate while the trustees managed the $300,000 in holdings that made up the corpus of the foundation. The establishment of the foundation and speculation about the size of Anderson's estate had been widely publicized, which in turn brought numerous proposals for how to spend the fortune. "As executors, we had been besieged with all kinds of crazy investment suggestions," said Thomas Anderson. "I remember opportunities to buy a circus, also a rodeo show—all kinds of opportunities to spend money foolishly—the list seemed endless. Of course, we had to take the time to carefully examine each one of them. They were all declined." Monroe Anderson was generous to his family; including a sister, Florie, who resided in the family hometown of Jackson; to his sisters-in-law, Burdine Clayton Anderson, Frank's widow, and his brother James's widow, who lived in Tuscaloosa, Alabama. He also left a generous inheritance to his nephews, the six sons of his brother Frank, and cousins and relatives in Colorado and Alabama. When the Internal Revenue Service finally declared that the $19 million destined for the foundation was indeed tax-exempt, the final processing of Anderson's will took place.[17]

On June 1, 1940, while the estate was going through a review by the IRS and probate, the Fulbright law firm made William B. Bates a named partner, and the firm became known as Fulbright, Crooker, Freeman & Bates. Later in the summer, on August 31, 1940, the two remaining trustees of the Anderson Foundation appointed Horace Morse Wilkins to succeed Monroe Anderson as trustee. Bates now became chairman and John Freeman became vice chairman. Wilkins had been a friend of Monroe Anderson and was highly respected in Houston's business community as an able banker. He was born January 9, 1885, to Capt. W. G. Wilkins and Eunice Lewis Wilkins in Brenham, Texas. His maternal grandfather was Col. Asa M. Lewis, who moved to Texas in 1838 or 1839 and served as an early member of the Republic of Texas Congress. Wilkins grew up in Brenham and then attended Texas A&M at College Station. He moved to Houston in 1902 and began a career in banking. In 1915 he and his brother, John A. Wilkins, with several associates, established the State Bank & Trust Company, which became the State National Bank of Houston in the 1930s. Horace Wilkins was president of the State National Bank of Houston, and William Bates and John Freeman both served as directors of the bank at the time.[18]

Early in 1941, after the IRS approved the foundation's status as a nonprofit charity and Anderson's will had been through probate, the estate then transferred $19 million to the foundation. The trustees approved a few modest grants, including $1,000 each to the Blue Bird Circle and the DePelchin Faith Home, and gifts to Memorial Hospital and the Crippled Children's Clinic. What began next was a series of events that took place across the state in Austin, Dallas, Houston, and Galveston, events that ultimately led to the M. D. Anderson Foundation's key

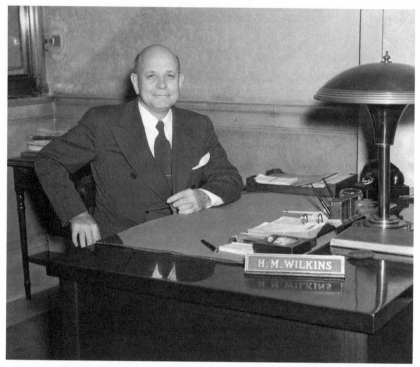

*Horace M. Wilkins. Courtesy of John P. McGovern Historical Collections and Research Center, Texas Medical Center Library.*

role in creating what since has become the largest medical center in the history of the world, the Texas Medical Center.[19]

As with many milestone moments in history, the string of events that brought about the birth of the Texas Medical Center has its origin deep in the past and, in this case, was in part instigated by one man's fierce determination to fight against a dreaded and deadly disease, cancer. In 1939 Arthur Cato, a druggist from Weatherford, Texas, first won election to the state legislature. Cato had lost both of his parents and members of his wife's family to cancer. On February 5, 1941, shortly after the next session of the Texas Legislature convened, Cato introduced House Bill 268, a bill to create a state cancer hospital.

Cancer was a disease that for much of its known history had a terrible stigma attached to it, a dreaded disease about which people did not talk in polite company. Thus, while people feared the deadly disease, little effort had been expended to learn its causes or develop new treatments. One of the first hopeful signs of change in the United States came about in the late nineteenth century. It began during the summer months of 1884 with the tragic news that former president Ulysses S. Grant had been diagnosed with throat cancer. Grant lived in New York City, and his valiant fight to complete his memoirs to provide for his family before succumbing to the disease captivated the public and brought a greater awareness of cancer. During the same year that Grant was diagnosed, several prominent residents of New York, including John Jacob Astor III, laid the cornerstone for the first hospital in the United States dedicated to providing care for cancer patients. The first phase of the New York Cancer Hospital opened in 1887, specifically to provide care for women. At the time, the treatment for cancer was limited to a few surgical procedures and mainly palliative efforts to make patients as comfortable as possible until they died. Morphine helped with the pain, and patients found distraction through carriage rides in nearby Central Park or at religious services in the hospital's chapel. Because cancer was so deadly and carried with it a terrible shame, fund-raising to support the hospital and its mission was exceedingly difficult. Around 1900 administrators changed the name to the General Memorial Hospital in an attempt to establish a fresh image. In the 1920s it became known as the General Memorial Hospital for the Treatment of Cancer and Allied Diseases. In 1936, the same year that Monroe Anderson created his foundation in Houston, John D. Rockefeller Jr. donated a tract of land on the east side of New York City, on York Avenue, adjacent to Cornell Medical College. Three years later, in 1939, Memorial Hospital opened on the site and the cancer hospital began the move into that facility. In 1940 Alfred P. Sloan and Charles F. Kettering, former executives of General Motors, established the Sloan-Kettering Institute, adjacent to the Memorial Hospital.[20]

In Texas, however, the fight against cancer took a somewhat different path. After 1900 medical doctors and some public health officials in the state began to take more interest in cancer. In 1914 the Texas Medical Association established a committee on cancer, making Texas the second state, after Pennsylvania, to create such a committee. In 1929 the state legislature authorized the creation of a cancer hospital in Dallas but did not appropriate funds, and the facility never opened.

As health care and sanitation continued to improve, people began living longer, and thus their bodies had more time to develop diseases, including cancer. By 1940 the death rate from cancer had continued increasing, to a point where the Committee on Cancer of the Texas Medical Association reported that the state needed to do more to provide treatment for the disease on behalf of the state's indigent patients. Now members of the Committee on Cancer were determined to press the issue once again. Dr. James M. Martin, who had been chair of the committee when the previous 1929 bill had passed, again took the lead, in concert with the State Department of Health, to draft a new bill. But Arthur Cato's bill was introduced first, much to Martin's surprise. Soon the two men began working together, along with Dr. John Spies, dean of the University of Texas Medical Branch in Galveston, to write one bill that could gain support from the state Senate and House of Representatives. The Texas Medical Association encouraged them to draft a bill that would associate the cancer hospital with the existing cancer program of the University of Texas. Spies worked with Cato on his original bill and then with the Texas Medical Association committee to rewrite the bill so that the new cancer hospital would be a part of the University of Texas and the Medical Branch in Galveston.[21]

Finally, on May 29, 1941, the Texas House of Representatives passed, by a vote of 85 to 39, Cato's House Bill 268 to establish the Texas State Cancer Hospital and the Division of Cancer Research. The House also appropriated $1.75 million to fund the new hospital. The Senate passed the bill but reduced the appropriation to $500,000. Still, the state had once again taken steps to create a state cancer hospital and this time had appropriated funds with which it could begin. On June 30, 1941, Governor W. Lee O'Daniel signed the bill into law.[22]

The legislation did not specify a location for the new hospital, leaving that decision up to University of Texas board of regents. This uncertainty led to some of the opposition to the measure that popped up around the state. Some in the legislature saw a cancer hospital as a hopeless waste of valuable funds and resources at a time when the country was preparing for its eventual involvement in World War II. Others saw its potential economic benefits and recognized the opportunities to advance medical research. Galvestonians expected the hospital would be located in their community, along with the University of

Texas Medical Branch. Politicians from Dallas lobbied to have it placed in their community, arguing that the 1929 legislation somehow set a precedent. And representatives from San Antonio noted that their city was more centrally located and therefore that the state's cancer hospital should be sited there. In the end, the board of regents would choose to put the cancer hospital in Houston, where it would become part of the legacy of M. D. Anderson.[23]

The probate process and IRS review of M. D. Anderson's will finally concluded in 1941, during the time that the legislature was in session. Dr. Frederick C. Elliott, dean of the Texas Dental College in Houston, saw a newspaper story about the foundation while he was on a trip to Austin. For years, Elliott had dreamed of creating a type of medical center in Houston. After a 1938 visit to the University of Pittsburgh, where he saw the school's magnificent, forty-two-story Cathedral of Learning, Elliott returned to Houston, inspired by the structure and believing that a similar building could house his medical center, including a medical school, nursing school, dental school, and hospital. He commissioned an architecture student to produce a preliminary drawing and had his dental students create plaster models of what he called the Memorial Center for Health Education. Elliott hoped that the new Anderson Foundation would be interested in his idea. At the time, the trustees were considering a few options but had not settled on any single idea.[24]

In fact, as John Freeman recalled years later, "We had nothing specific in mind at the start. We had cast about to see where and in what manner we might best put this resource to work. Two or three things developed that led us to consider health as a matter that needed attention." The trustees began considering an idea to develop a hospital for what they called "the white collar man." At that time, most hospitals served either the very rich or the very poor, and the average middle-income, working-class people were left with few options for hospital care. Baker Memorial Pavilion of Massachusetts General Hospital provided such services and had seemed to Freeman a model that the Anderson Foundation could emulate in Houston. The hospital established fees when a patient entered that covered medical treatment, hospital expenses, and medication. "If you were there for two weeks or for three months, the price was the same," said Freeman. "You had to qualify to be eligible to go into that Baker Memorial Pavilion, but that's the way it was operated. We were looking at that idea when the Texas Legislature authorized a cancer research hospital for the state in 1941. That took our attention immediately, and we moved over to that idea and away from what we had been thinking."[25]

William B. Bates later stated in an interview that he saw an article in the newspaper about the legislature passing the bill to create a state cancer hospital and appropriating $500,000 for the University of Texas to begin the project. The legislation made it possible for the university to receive private gifts for the hospital as well. "After consultation with Mr. Freeman and Mr. Wilkins, we all decided it would be a wonderful thing," said Bates. "They could have that hospital in Houston, and we would be glad to make some donation." Bates contacted Dr. John Spies and arranged a meeting at his home in Houston. Following this initial session, several meetings took place that at times included Dr. Homer Rainey, president of the University of Texas, and members of the board of regents. These early conversations were often exploratory and informal, with several of them taking place on the back porch of Bates's home on Brentwood Drive. "There was a ceiling fan there to assist the prevailing breeze," said Freeman. "Not much air conditioning then, you know—and it was just a comfortable situation for relaxed conversation. Colonel Bates, Mr. Wilkins, and I had met there frequently after hours to discuss the affairs of the Anderson Foundation, and so it was just natural to invite these men to join us there from time to time."[26]

During their first meeting, Bates told Spies that he believed the cancer hospital should be located in a city larger than Galveston, but he was also concerned about making sure that Houston was the right place. In an account years later, Bates wrote: "We explained to the university people that we didn't want to induce them to locate the cancer hospital in Houston if it wasn't the proper place. We thought it was. Houston was Texas's largest city, close to Galveston and the medical school and all." Many Houstonians believed that the state had erred in locating the Medical Branch in Galveston. In 1923 brothers Mike and Will Hogg, businessmen and civic leaders, purchased 134 acres south of Hermann Hospital through their Varner Realty company, all with the hope of enticing the University of Texas to move the Medical Branch from Galveston to this plot of land in Houston. Once it became clear that this would not happen, they sold the land to the city at cost. In 1941, while engaged in an ugly fight to save his job as dean of the Medical Branch, Spies secretly aspired to move it to Houston. According to Frederick Elliott, "Since the cancer hospital was to be built in Houston he [Spies] wanted the dental school [Texas Dental College] also to continue to operate in Houston. It was his plan to use these two institutions that were planned for Houston as a springboard in his desire to move the Medical Branch from Galveston to Houston." Spies's plans never materialized and, caught up in a nasty struggle to save his job, there was little time for him to fight against the powerful interests in Galveston that would never accept losing "their" medical school.[27]

Discussions between the trustees of the Anderson Foundation and the University of Texas continued in Austin and on Bates's back porch. Finally, on March 10, 1942, the Anderson trustees drew up a formal agreement. As Freeman later recalled: "We worked out an arrangement whereby the Foundation agreed that if the University of Texas would establish the cancer research hospital in Houston and call it the M. D. Anderson Hospital, we would furnish $500,000 to match the sum appropriated by the legislature, and we would provide twenty acres of ground at an appropriate place in Houston on which to build the hospital." The proposed agreement called for the University of Texas to maintain administrative and managerial control over the hospital. The Anderson Foundation would not have any responsibility for managing the facility or providing funds for its operational needs.[28]

Now that the Anderson Foundation trustees had submitted a formal proposal to the University of Texas, it was up to the board of regents to make the final decision on whether to accept the offer and choose Houston as the site of the state's new cancer hospital. Their approval of the agreement would ensure the legacy of Monroe D. Anderson far beyond the imagination of his trusted friends who now ran his foundation. Years later, Bates paid tribute to his client and friend:

> Mr. Anderson lived simply and unostentatiously. He was guided by a few simple basic principles which probably were responsible for the greatness he attained. To him it was axiomatic that neither an individual nor people as a whole can ever be happy or prosper without hard work, thrift, and self-denial; that laziness and profligate spending inevitably lead to misery, poverty,

and sorrow. He did not believe in personal charity for the individual, except for the handicapped and afflicted. In his opinion, an individual sound in body and mind who sought or accepted charity was not worthy of it. But he did believe in improving the opportunity of the unfortunate to help himself, and in giving remedial relief and comfort to the sick and helpless. These simple rules of conduct and thought guided his life. Thus he created his great fortune and was motivated to dedicate his wealth for the benevolent purposes so strikingly set forth in the trust indenture of the M. D. Anderson Foundation. . . . The M. D. Anderson Foundation is Mr. Anderson's great gift and legacy to the residents of this community."[29]

Although they believed the prospects for locating the hospital in Houston were good, the Anderson Foundation trustees needed to find a temporary home for the cancer hospital to help secure the deal. And the University of Texas had to find a qualified person to step into a leadership role as an interim director in order to ensure that the hospital would become a reality. With World War II now raging and the United States fully involved, both human resources and materials for construction would soon be in short supply. The messy business regarding the dean of the Medical Branch was taking a new turn, and in many ways it was not far-fetched to wonder if Arthur Cato's dream of a state cancer hospital would suffer the same fate as the effort of 1929. But the Anderson trustees were determined that the hospital named for their benefactor would succeed. They had ample resources, broad-based support from Houston's business and civic leaders, and, in the end, destiny on their side.

# Chapter 5

## *Bold Vision*

### First Steps toward Building a Medical Center

During the spring of 1942, while the University of Texas board of regents considered the Anderson Foundation's proposal to locate the state's new cancer hospital in Houston, the Anderson Foundation trustees began to think seriously about also creating a major medical center. Dr. E. W. Bertner, one of the city's leading physicians, had long dreamed of creating such a center, a dream also shared by the city's highest-ranking educator in the health fields, Dr. Frederick C. Elliott, dean of the Texas Dental College. Both of these men were acquainted with the Anderson Foundation trustees and took leading roles as the trustees moved to forge serious plans for their medical center. They knew that the center would need hospitals, a medical school, and more. As they continued to develop their initial plans, their first order of business was to find a temporary location for the cancer hospital and a qualified physician to serve as administrator. Once the cancer hospital was under way, they could look at filling the other needs for the future medical center.

By early 1942, with the United States fully involved in World War II, new construction unrelated to the war effort was prohibited, and many items were subject to rationing in order to direct needed resources to support the troops. This meant that the Anderson trustees would have to find an existing building that could be adapted as a cancer hospital, one that would be serviceable until after the war ended and perhaps well beyond, when construction of a new facility could begin. Finding a suitable location might provide additional assurance for the University of Texas to a point where the regents would select Houston over other Texas cities in what had become a fierce competition for the new cancer hospital. One of the Houston sites that held promise was the old, original, 150-bed Jefferson Davis Hospital, built in 1924 at 1101 Elder Street. A new hospital had opened in 1938, and the original building sat empty. "We looked all through that old building," trustee William Bates recalled years later. "It was a wreck. We decided it would cost too much to remodel it." The trustees then learned that the late Capt. James A. Baker, a prominent Houston attorney who had died several months earlier, had given his estate to the Rice Institute. The estate, known as The Oaks, was located near downtown at 2310 Baldwin Street. It included a large home, stables, and small outbuildings situated on about six acres of beautifully landscaped grounds. Baker had been a friend of and Houston attorney for businessman William Marsh Rice. After Rice was murdered in New York in 1900, Baker helped to convict the murderers, Rice's valet and his New York City attorney, and prevented a fraudulent will from being probated. Thus, he helped ensure that the Rice fortune, which had grown to almost $10 million, would be directed as Rice intended to establish the Rice Institute in Houston. Baker was the founding chairman of the university's board of trustees and served on the board from the time of its initial charter in 1891 until his death on August 2, 1941. When the Rice trustees concluded that they had no practical use for the Baker estate, they offered to sell it to the Anderson Foundation for $68,000. The Anderson trustees determined that this was a reasonable price, purchased the property on May 16, 1942, and then turned it over to the University of Texas as a temporary site for the new M. D. Anderson Hospital for Cancer Research. In contrast to Jefferson Davis Hospital, the buildings of the Baker estate were in excellent condition, and the location, just south of downtown, provided convenient access for patients and doctors. Historian James S. Olson, in his history of the M. D. Anderson Cancer Center, described the grounds as having "carefully manicured shrubs, broad stretches of mowed and edged grass, and large cypress trees tangled in wisteria. The main residence, its brown brick exterior draped in thick ivy, had a basement and two other floors. Behind the main residence, the two-story stable and carriage house could be refitted for research laboratories."[1]

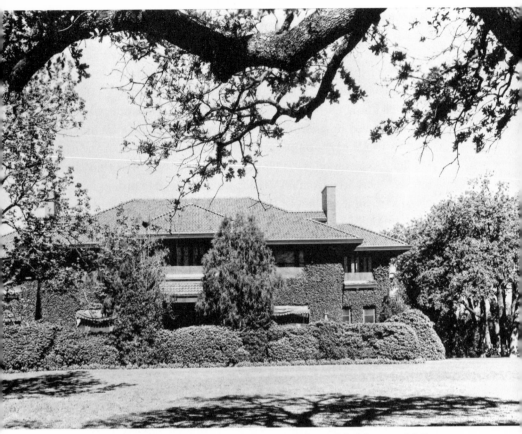

*Main house at The Oaks, former estate of Capt. James A. Baker and first home to M. D. Anderson Hospital for Cancer Research. Courtesy of John P. McGovern Historical Collections and Research Center, Texas Medical Center Library.*

Now that the proposed cancer hospital had a temporary home available in Houston and with all indications being that the University of Texas board of regents would approve the Anderson Foundation's proposal, the next priority was to find the right person with the energy, enthusiasm, credentials, and leadership skills to get the new hospital organized and opened. The director would have to be a medical doctor with a fine reputation and also a passion for fighting cancer. Some initially thought that Dr. John Spies, the dean of the University of Texas Medical Branch in Galveston, might be tapped for this responsibility. But on June 5, 1942, the university fired him. Spies had been embroiled in a bitter and divisive controversy almost since his arrival at UTMB in January 1939, and by the spring of 1942 the regents had had enough.[2]

In the meantime, a candidate had already emerged who had the unique capabilities to launch the new cancer hospital, at least on an interim basis until after the war. Houston physician Ernst W. "Bill" Bertner was well known in Texas medical circles and well connected politically, having served in a number of high-profile positions, including president of the Harris County Medical Society and president of the Texas Medical Association. Dr. Elliott recalled in his memoir that shortly after Spies was fired from UTMB, Dr. Judson Taylor, a prominent Houston physician, invited Elliot to lunch where he expressed his concerns that an acting director might be appointed to run the cancer hospital who did not share their ideas about creating a full-fledged medical center in Houston. Already, behind the scenes, UT president Homer Rainey had been thinking of consolidating all of the university's medical schools on the main campus in Austin. At Taylor's suggestion, Elliott, who was acquainted with Rainey, recommended Bertner to be the interim director of the university's new cancer hospital. Members of Houston's business community also jumped on the bandwagon for Bertner. The board of regents saw that he was the obvious and best choice and appointed him as acting director of the cancer hospital beginning August 1, 1942. The university offered Bertner a salary of $10,000, but he graciously declined and instead asked that the funds be applied to the operating account to help get the new hospital opened.[3]

Bertner believed strongly in the mission of the cancer hospital and was also an early proponent of creating a medical center in Houston. Indeed, if there is one physician who could be viewed as being the "father" of the Texas Medical Center, that person would be Dr. Ernst W. Bertner. His leadership gave shape to the Texas Medical Center and had a lasting impact on how it developed over time. E. W. "Billy" Bertner, as he was known to his friends, was born in the West Texas railroad boomtown of Colorado City on August 18, 1889. He was said to have been a rambunctious child and proved to be a handful for his father, Gus, a German immigrant, and his mother, Anna Miller Bertner. Gus Bertner was a barber by trade and made a good living in Colorado City. But as the community's fortunes and population faded in the early 1900s, Bertner began a new career as a regional sales representative for New York Life

Insurance. The very personable Gus Bertner thrived in the new position and in later years, by the 1930s, was frequently a member of the "Million Dollar Club," which honored salesmen who earned over a million dollars annually for the company.[4]

As Ernst Bertner grew into his teenage years, Gus saw that his only son needed a firmer, more structured environment, and in 1904 he sent the young man to the New Mexico Military Institute for high school. Bertner was to be part of the class of 1908 but for unknown reasons left school after the spring term in 1906 and returned to Colorado City, where his father then bought a drugstore for him to manage. Bertner was a gregarious, affable, fun-loving young man, and the drugstore was a pleasant environment for him. But during the next year, as he learned the drugstore business, a new law in Texas cast a shadow over the family's future in Colorado City. Texas governor Thomas M. Campbell, a self-proclaimed reformer, supported legislation to impose strong supervision over non-Texas life insurance companies. In 1907 the legislature enacted the Robertson Insurance Law, a compulsory investment law that put an end to the practice of out-of-state insurance companies making large profits but not investing in the state. The law required all out-of-state life insurance companies doing business in Texas to invest 75 percent of their Texas reserves in Texas securities to help guarantee Texas businesses and loans. Rather than adhere to what they viewed as restrictive requirements of the new law, most large life insurance companies—New York Life included—relocated to other states. After almost two decades of living in Colorado City, Gus and Anna were also forced to relocate. They chose to move to Little Rock, Arkansas, where they would spend the remainder of their lives. [5]

During his first year of managing the drugstore, Ernst Bertner had developed an interest in pharmaceuticals and how they worked to provide relief for patients. In 1907 he decided to move beyond clerking in his drugstore and develop expertise in the field of pharmacology. In September Bertner left Colorado City to attend the University of Texas School of Pharmacy in Galveston. Responding to the urging of a faculty member and family friend after he arrived, Bertner changed course and decided to seek a degree in medicine. But his gregarious nature found the temptations of life in the wide-open city of Galveston to be very distracting. Near the end of the fall term, Gus Bertner became concerned about both his son's physical health and his academic progress. He wrote to the dean, Dr. William S. Carter, and asked, "Please be so kind and inform me how [Ernst] is getting along and what ailment he has." Carter sent a reply stating that young Bertner's health was fine but also included a tactful reproach of his indulgent father, hinting of what was to come. "It is impossible to give a definite statement as to his work before the results of [fall] examinations are reported to us in January," Carter wrote. He then added, "It requires constant attention and effort on the part of the student to do the work that is required in this school, and they should not be furnished with too large an allowance [if] they are expected to be successful."[6]

While home for Christmas break in 1907, Ernst received a telegram from Dean Carter with the disheartening news that he was passing only two out of six subjects. Carter suggested that the young medical student resign. After days of reflecting on his future, Ernst concluded that he, in fact, really did want to become a medical doctor. On the day after Christmas, a deeply shaken young Bertner boarded a train for Galveston to plead with the dean for a second chance. The sincerity and forcefulness of Bertner's appeal inspired Carter to reconsider the young man's fate. But despite his inclination to give Bertner another chance, Carter left the final decision to the university's board of regents. At a special hearing, Bertner successfully persuaded the regents to give him a reprieve. He thus began his second term of medical school on probation, in which he had to meet certain requisites or "conditions" in order to continue. While the Dean's Office record for 1908 lists Bertner under "Freshman Conditioned" for biology, physics, and embryology, it is uncertain what specific requirements he had to fulfill. It is also unclear if these or other arrangements were made regarding the other courses Bertner was failing. Nevertheless, Bertner's newly found focus and determination to succeed served him well, and he avoided the "Condition List" throughout the remainder of medical school.[7]

In 1911 he received his medical degree and left for internship and residency at Willard Parker Hospital, St. Vincent's Hospital, and the Manhattan Maternity Hospital in New York City. Here he trained under the guidance of nationally renowned surgeons E. L. Keyes and George D. Stewart, learning the latest advances in surgery, therapeutics, and research. On one of these occasions, as was common in those days, Dr.

Stewart asked his intern to serve as the anesthetist for a patient from Houston. Bertner did so and later checked up on the patient, Jesse H. Jones, as he convalesced. Jones enjoyed the visits from the young intern and made an offer that was hard for Bertner to resist. Jones was building a new Rice Hotel in downtown Houston, on the site of the old hotel that he acquired from Rice University and had demolished in 1911. The beautiful new $3 million, 500-room hotel was nearing completion and was set to open in the spring 1913. He needed a house physician on staff and saw in Bertner a very capable, personable young physician—seemingly a perfect match. Bertner was in search of a community where he could establish himself and open a medical practice after he completed his residency training. Little Rock, Arkansas, where his father had moved the family by this time, did not have long-term appeal. Houston, on the other hand, was abounding in opportunity in the years following the discovery of oil at Spindletop in 1901. It was the place to be for anyone with a passion for life and a desire to succeed. At Jones's invitation, Bertner visited Houston and, like many other transplanted residents, saw the city as a place of tremendous opportunity. In July 1913 he moved to Houston and into the Rice Hotel, where he would reside for the rest of his life. He and Jesse Jones became very close, lifelong friends.[8]

Bertner opened an office at 412 Carter Building, where he established his medical practice. He remained in Houston from 1913 until late April or early May 1917, when he became the first Houston physician to enlist in the Army Medical Corps during World War I. Upon arriving in Europe, Lt. Bertner served first with the British army and later joined the American Expeditionary Force (AEF) when it arrived in France. From February 1918 to March 1919 Bertner served on the staff of Gen. John J. Pershing as an aide to Col. Hugh H. Young. Dr. Young, a Texan born in San Antonio, was world renowned in his field, had been chairman of urology at the Johns Hopkins School of Medicine and head of the Brady Urological Institute, and now served as director of the urology division of the AEF. Bertner also served with Maj. E. L. Keyes Jr., a highly regarded urologist under whom he had trained as an intern in New York.[9]

Captain Bertner was discharged from the Army Medical Corps on April 19, 1919, at Camp Dix, New Jersey, and returned to Houston to resume his medical practice. His military service opened his mind to new ideas and drove home some important lessons for Bertner. First, he had witnessed how a team of doctors working together could provide comprehensive medical care—in this case, in the battlefield hospitals—having a significant impact on the outcomes for the patients. He would carry this lesson home and began considering how it might apply in domestic medical practice. Second, Bertner realized that he needed more training and in 1921 took a leave from his practice and accepted a residency at Johns Hopkins, where he would study surgery, urology, and gynecology. He worked six months with his friend Dr. Hugh Young and six months with Dr. Thomas Cullen in what has been described as "a pivotal year in his career." Hugh Young was the recognized leader of urology in the United States and an authority on neoplasms (tumors) in this field. Thomas Cullen, chairman of gynecology at Hopkins, was a renowned authority on gynecologic cancer and an early leader in the national campaign for cancer control. Under Cullen, Bertner gained experience treating uterine, cervical, ovarian, and breast cancer and soon became a leader in the fight against the dread disease.[10]

In May 1922 Bertner again returned to Houston and resumed his practice. The yearlong fellowship had a profound impact on him. He had become a more competent physician and had also developed an intense interest in cancer. In addition, Bertner saw firsthand the benefits of bringing together all aspects of medical education and patient care in a large medical center. He observed how the very best minds and skills could come together for improved patient care, teaching of students, and research. All of this energized Bertner, and the pace of his life quickened as he began to take on more professional responsibility. First, in October 1922, he became a Fellow in the Texas Surgical Society. His personal life changed in a wonderful way during this time when on November 30, 1922, he married Julia Williams in St. Louis, Missouri. The couple settled in Houston, in the Rice Hotel, where they lived for their entire married life. Bertner's medical practice continued to grow during the ensuing years and so did his leadership role in the community. In 1933 Bertner became president of the Harris County Medical Society, and in 1935 he became president of the Postgraduate Medical Assembly, president of the Texas Surgical Society, Chief of Staff at Hermann Hospital, and served on several committees of the Texas Medical Association.

*Dr. Ernst W. Bertner as a young man. Courtesy of E. W. and Julia Bertner Family.*

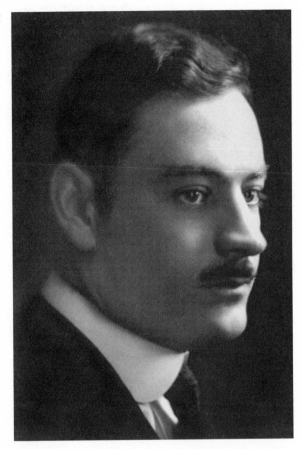

In 1937, Ernst and Julia Bertner took time off for a two-month trip to Europe with close friends Dr. and Mrs. Robert A. Johnston. Years later, Julia Bertner recalled how they visited nearly every major hospital—the best medical centers in Europe—in order for her husband to learn their best practices, hoping to incorporate them one day and fulfill his dream of establishing a medical center in Houston. Continuing his leadership in the medical profession, in 1938 Bertner was named president-elect of the Texas Medical Association and in 1939 became president. As president of the TMA, Bertner was known as "a vigorous defender of the private practice of medicine."[11]

Bertner did not take an active role in the initial planning for the cancer center and generally supported Spies's ideas about it. But once the Anderson Foundation took the lead in the effort to locate the hospital

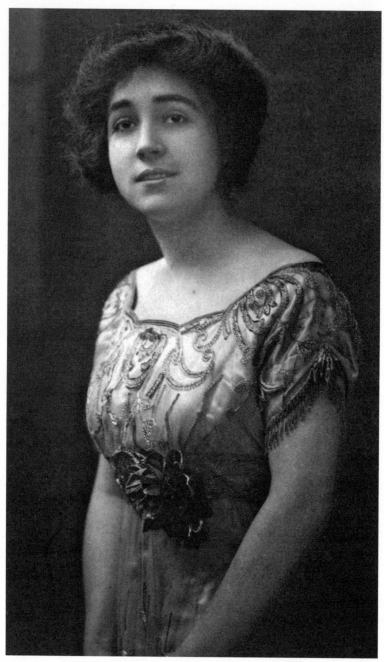

*Julia Williams Bertner. Courtesy of E. W. and Julia Bertner Family.*

in Houston, the trustees recruited Bertner to their cause. Years later, John H. Freeman reflected that he and his wife lived in an apartment on the same floor of the Rice Hotel as the Bertners and had many opportunities to visit back and forth. "Colonel Bates, Mr. Wilkins, and I were close friends, and we often found ourselves up there on the top floor of the Rice Hotel, consulting with Dr. Bertner," said Freeman. He emphasized the significance of those conversations for the cancer hospital and the Texas Medical Center, noting, "The Anderson Foundation Trustees had no medical training, no medical experience at all. We wouldn't have known how to proceed if it hadn't been for Dr. Bertner's help and advice."[12]

Although the regents had not formally approved the proposal to locate the new cancer hospital in Houston, the Anderson Foundation's gift of The Oaks as a temporary site likely helped secure the deal. On August 8, 1942, one week after Dr. Bertner's position as acting director of the cancer hospital became effective, the University of Texas board of regents officially accepted the Anderson Foundation's proposal. Once the board of regents formally agreed to locate the new cancer hospital in Houston, the Anderson Foundation trustees then made the commitment to create a medical center in the city. "When we took the cancer hospital in hand, we then made up our minds that we would try to put a [medical] center in here," said John Freeman. "We didn't envision anything like it is now, of course, but we wanted to put in a sizeable center." The Anderson trustees even went so far as to suggest that the University of Texas consider opening a branch of its Galveston medical school in Houston. They recognized that to have a major medical center, Houston would need educational, research, and library facilities, along with hospitals. Frederick Elliott related that when he heard the news that the state cancer hospital would be located in Houston, he saw an opportunity for a different kind of medical center than his original concept. In his memoirs he wrote, "The Memorial Center for Health Education, as such, was shelved by us at the dental college," and he began a campaign to have the University of Texas incorporate the Texas Dental College into its system to be a part of this future medical center.[13]

Several weeks later, on September 25, 1942, the board of regents formally agreed to name the hospital the M. D. Anderson Hospital for Cancer Research of the University of Texas. An enthusiastic Bertner focused his energy on opening the hospital and on laying the ground-work to create a medical center. He hired architects to develop plans for renovations of the existing buildings and hoped to gain government approval for a one-story clinic building that would be adjacent to the main house, which then would be converted to an office and staff building. The basement became the temporary location for the X-ray equipment, and the stables were converted into research laboratories. Dr. Chauncey Leake, the new dean of the University of Texas Medical Branch in Galveston, also presided over the university's new Houston cancer hospital. He agreed to loan faculty members to the fledgling hospital and also provided the services of John Musgrove, a business manager whose administrative skills, stamina, and willingness to do almost any task to help build the hospital were crucial to the effort for many years.[14]

As 1942 quickly rolled into 1943, Bertner worked feverishly to convert The Oaks into a cancer hospital. During the coming months, he managed to build the clinic and arranged to lease twenty-two beds from Hermann Hospital for cancer patients and six beds from the Houston Negro Hospital to accommodate black patients during what remained an era of racial segregation. The M. D. Anderson Foundation had a key role in facilitating the use of hospital beds at Hermann Hospital by agreeing to provide funds for a new facility for the hospital's interns and residents. Because of the war effort and the ban on new major construction, even small jobs like those that Bertner proposed were extremely difficult to complete. Construction materials and craftsmen were scarce, prices unstable, and state officials reluctant to provide additional funding. Still, Bertner, along with the indispensable John Musgrove, persisted in efforts to convert the estate into a serviceable cancer hospital. On June 26, 1943, the board of regents announced the appointment of the first clinical staff of the cancer hospital, an all-star lineup of prominent physicians and surgeons in Houston: Drs. Joe B. Foster, John H. Foster, E. L. Goar, Herbert T. Hayes, Robert A. Johnston, Ben Weems Turner, James Greenwood, C. M. Griswold, M. D. Levy, David Greer, Frederick C. Elliott, Judson Taylor, John H. Poster, and E. William Bertner. Bertner had selected the staff and recommended them to the board of regents. But several months would pass before the hospital could begin receiving patients. During this hectic period, Bertner, Elliott, and the Anderson Foundation trustees continued to work on plans to develop a full-fledged medical center and devoted considerable time in discussions with officials from the University of Texas.[15]

While Bertner worked to transform the Baker estate into a fully functional cancer hospital, Dr. Frederick C. Elliott, dean of the privately held Texas Dental College, saw an opportunity to establish a similar affiliation with the University of Texas. With a renewed sense of purpose, Elliott resumed his efforts to secure a university affiliation and began a campaign to make the dental school a part of the University of Texas

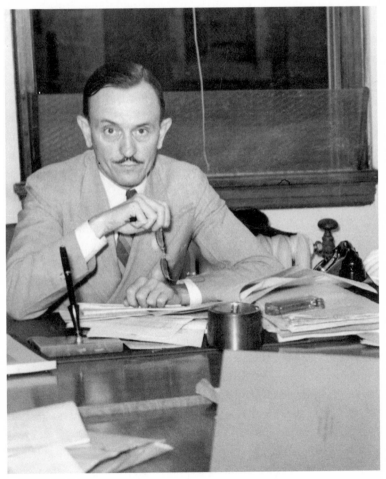

*Dr. Frederick C. Elliott, dean of the Texas Dental College. Courtesy of John P. McGovern Historical Collections and Research Center, Texas Medical Center Library.*

system. In the waning months of 1942, he launched a publicity drive to gain support for the move from throughout the state. By the time the next legislative session began in January 1943, Elliott was confident that his goal of bringing the Texas Dental College into an affiliation with the university would be successful. The college had opened in 1903 as a private, for-profit institution and was later converted to a nonprofit school by a group of philanthropic, public-spirited dentists. The Houston school and Baylor Dental College in Dallas were the only institutions for the training of dentists in Texas. Elliott had been recruited as dean of the college in 1932 in an attempt to save the struggling institution from going under. During his tenure as dean, the school emerged from debt and had attained a value of about $150,000. Now Elliott proposed to donate its entire property and facilities to the state of Texas if the legislature would authorize the University of Texas to take over the college, making it the dental branch of the university. The Houston Chamber of Commerce supported Elliott's plan, and the M. D. Anderson Foundation agreed to provide land for a permanent home for the dental branch and also proposed a donation of $500,000 to help meet the cost of a permanent building. The legislature passed House Bill 279 and its companion bill in the Senate in May 1943.[16]

In this way, the Texas Dental College would become one of the cornerstone institutions in the fledgling medical center. Elliott, as dean of the dental college, also was Houston's highest-ranking educator in the health fields and had been an advocate for a medical center for several years. He served on many public health committees and first became acquainted with Colonel Bates when both men served on the Chamber of Commerce. "Dr. Elliott was very active in health matters," Bates recalled later. "He served ably as chairman of the Chamber's Health Committee. I soon found out he knew more about public health than many doctors I had come in contact with, although his field was dentistry." Thus, his background in higher education as professor of dentistry and dean offered an important perspective as trustees of the Anderson Foundation and others continued to make plans for a medical center. John H. Freeman later recalled, "We were encouraged by the work of Dr. Fred Elliott and others to bring Texas Dental College, located here in Houston, into the University of Texas System. That turned out to be an important factor in the creation of the medical center."[17]

The bill introduced by Arthur Cato and passed by the state legislature in 1941 set in motion a series of events that culminated with the
University of Texas board of regents' decision to accept the bold offer
from the Anderson Foundation and locate the cancer hospital in Houston. This move by the Anderson Foundation trustees, William B. Bates,
John H. Freeman, and Horace M. Wilkins, proved to be the most significant development in the creation of the Texas Medical Center, the
catalyst that would result in Houston ultimately becoming the home to
the largest medical complex in human history. The cancer hospital became the first institution of what would develop into the Texas Medical
Center and would ensure that the legacy of Monroe D. Anderson would
extend far beyond the imagination of the trusted friends who now ran
his foundation.

# Chapter 6

## *Building Blocks*

### Baylor University College of Medicine

During the months that E. W. Bertner was scrambling to open the cancer hospital and Frederick Elliott was busy lobbying the state legislature to assimilate the Texas Dental College into the University of Texas, a storm was building in Dallas over Baylor University College of Medicine. The events that occurred in North Texas during 1942–43 would have a major impact on the hoped-for medical center in Houston and, for a time, created a major drama in the state. While it is not the purpose of this book to present a history of Baylor College of Medicine, it is important to take a brief look at the events of 1942–43 to see the pivotal role of the M. D. Anderson Foundation in facilitating the introduction of a medical school in Houston and in creating the beginnings of what would one day become the Texas Medical Center.[1]

In 1900 a small group of Dallas-area physicians and other local citizens established a medical school that they named the University of Dallas Medical Department. The fact that there was no such entity as the University of Dallas seemed not to bother these ambitious founders, and the school opened on October 30, 1900. Within three years they established an alliance with Baylor University in Waco and changed the name of their school to Baylor University College of Medicine. During the next two decades, the medical school struggled financially, but in 1920, it received a grant from the General Education Board of New York. Then Baylor University's board of trustees pledged $50,000 a year in matching funds for the medical school, and it seemed that its financial stability was assured. But this confidence proved to be misplaced and, as the years passed and the country suffered through the Great Depression of the 1930s, the medical school received little of the promised support from its distant parent institution in Waco. By 1938, the financial situation had reached a point that some supporters, including the former dean, Dr. Edward H. Cary, believed it threatened the very existence of the medical school. The buildings were inadequate, and the school had a faculty of only eighteen instructors, relying mainly on physicians who practiced in the greater Dallas area to serve as volunteer faculty.[2]

Cary had joined the faculty of the University of Dallas Medical Department in January 1902. Just three months later, in April, the school's trustees appointed Cary as dean, a position that he held for the next seventeen years. In 1920 Cary resigned to pursue other activities and also to serve as president of the American Medical Association. He was succeeded as dean by Dr. Walter H. Moursund, a specialist in pathology and bacteriology who had been on the faculty since 1911. Moursund worked in many roles at Baylor, including professor of physiology, pathology, clinical pathology, bacteriology, and hygiene. He also served as secretary and registrar, acting dean, and ultimately as dean from 1923 until he retired in 1953. Despite the challenges of the era and the Great Depression of the 1930s, Baylor University College of Medicine continued to train students to become physicians. But by 1938, former dean Edward Cary had come to believe that his beloved medical school was in very dire straits and soon would be forced to close. In an attempt to attract more funding and save the school, he decided to act. In 1939 he helped to charter the Southwestern Medical Foundation in order to raise funds, provide updated facilities near the new Parkland Hospital in Dallas, and essentially take over the medical school operations from the sectarian control of the Baptist trustees and administrators in Waco. Cary believed that the medical school would never gain the level of financial support it needed in Dallas as long as it was controlled by the Baylor University trustees as a Baptist institution.

In March 1942 Cary proposed a merger of Baylor University College of Medicine and the Southwestern Medical Foundation, a union that was tantamount to a hostile takeover of the medical school. The terms of the merger agreement stated that the Southwestern Medical Foundation would provide twenty acres of land and a minimum of $1 million, of which at least $750,000 would be for new quarters for the medical and dental colleges, to be completed within two years of the lifting of wartime construction priorities. In addition, beginning with the 1942 academic term, the foundation was to furnish a minimum of $20,000 per year in additional financial support for the medical college. The administrative structure would change in that the medical college was to be governed by an administrative committee consisting of three members appointed by the foundation and two members appointed by the trustees of Baylor University. Although Baylor could overrule the administrative committee, the foundation, which held ownership of the property and new buildings, could end the agreement and take over all the facilities of the medical school. Cary quickly won public support for the merger and, more importantly, support from the city's doctors who constituted the school's volunteer clinical faculty. Behind this support was the implication that if the merger failed, the doctors would resign as faculty and the school would not be able to continue. World War II was raging, and a shortage of physicians was already felt in the nation's medical schools. In addition, fund-raising essentially ceased as all resources now were aimed to support the war effort. Under this pressure, all but three Baylor University trustees signed the agreement proffered by the Southwestern Medical Foundation on June 23, 1942.[3]

Walter H. Moursund, dean of the medical school at the time, later wrote in his book, *A History of Baylor University College of Medicine, 1900–1953*, "The restrictions of this agreement made many pause to wonder if the Southwestern Medical Foundation wanted Baylor University College of Medicine in its medical center or if the foundation wanted to operate its own medical college in the center." Moursund expressed the suspicions of many at Baylor and noted that other medical colleges had become "an integral part of medical centers without sacrificing their university affiliation or their administrative control. Yet, this sacrifice of affiliation and control in return for promised financial aid and new buildings seemed, to some, to be inherent terms of this agreement."[4]

In his book Moursund refuted much of Cary's criticism regarding the financial condition of the medical school and the alleged fund-raising handicaps caused by its affiliation with the Baptist-owned Baylor University. He also stated that from the Southwestern Medical

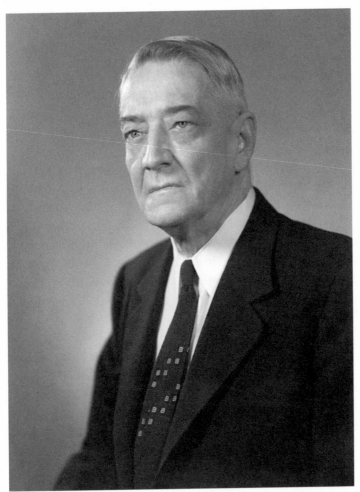

*Dr. Walter H. Moursund, dean of Baylor University College of Medicine.*
*Courtesy of John P. McGovern Historical Collections and Research Center,*
*Texas Medical Center Library.*

Foundation's inception, it had not raised the endowment funds it had
promised nor did it provide any direct financial assistance to the medical school. Moursund asserted that the medical college was in no worse
financial shape in 1942 than it had been in previous years. He took particular issue with Cary's allegations that the school's sectarian nature
inhibited fund-raising and brought about interference and meddling by
the Baptist trustees:

There was much discussion on the part of Dr. Cary, dean emeritus of the college and president of the foundation, and other supporters of the foundation, that the college was handicapped and could not obtain financial support, because it was sectarian in conduct and control. It is hard to believe that those who held this view and tried to make capital of it had not known that throughout the years past the college of medicine had been operated and conducted without any sectarian or denominational domination or interference. The writer, a Presbyterian, had been dean of the college for the past twenty years. Throughout the years the medical college had received outside financial aid. Several grants from the Rockefeller Foundation had been received as well as aid from other organizations and from individuals. The need for funds in 1942 was not desperate, but the trustees of Baylor University and the administrators of the medical college wanted the college to continue its progress and growth.[5]

About two weeks after the Baylor University trustees signed the merger agreement, on July 7, 1942, the executive board of the General Baptist Convention of Texas voted to approve the agreement with the Southwestern Medical Foundation. The full Texas Baptist Convention then approved it in November. But from the moment the Baylor trustees signed the agreement, the three trustees who had voted against it, Carr P. Collins, D. K. Martin, and H. L. Kokernot, became increasingly more determined not to let the medical school fall under the control of the foundation. As Martin recalled years later, "Every Baylor Trustee, except H. L. Kokernot, Carr P. Collins, and the writer, D. K. Martin, voted for the Merger Agreement. Carr Collins made the best speech of his life against the Merger. When the Merger was voted, Carr Collins resigned from the Baylor Board in protest." Shortly after the trustees voted on the agreement, Collins, Kokernot, and Martin went to the ranch of Kokernot's son-in-law, Gunter Hardy, in San Antonio. For the next three days, they enjoyed the outdoors and vented their frustration over the merger vote by riding horses, fishing, and also talking about the vote. According to Martin, they concluded that this agreement could not be allowed to stand and that Baylor had only three choices regarding the College of Medicine: give the school away, close the school, or move the school someplace else, although they admitted "to where and how we knew not." Martin stated that just before dinner, on the third day that they were at the ranch, one of them suggested that the trustees of the M. D. Anderson Foundation might make it possible for Baylor to move the College of Medicine to Houston. The three men agreed to follow through on that suggestion, and, as Martin recalled it, "Kokernot and Carr took me to San Antonio that night and I caught a midnight train to Houston."[6]

In an unusual twist of irony, it turned out that Clarence Fulbright was the attorney who wrote the charter to establish the Southwestern Medical Foundation in 1939. He and D. K. Martin had been roommates at Baylor during their college days and remained good friends until Fulbright died in 1940. As Martin stated, "Fulbright had no thought in the world but to render service to Baylor. He never dreamed that later the Foundation, under the Charter he had prepared, would seek to control Baylor College of Medicine." Martin had met William Bates and John Freeman years before through Fulbright. He knew Freeman better, so he set up a meeting with him. After a lengthy discussion, Martin told Freeman that he, Kokernot, and Collins wondered whether the Anderson Foundation trustees would be interested in helping Baylor move its College of Medicine to Houston. "I don't know whether you can move Baylor College of Medicine to Houston or not," Freeman told Martin. "And of course I am just one trustee, but you have just mentioned something that appeals to me more as a trustee of the Anderson Foundation than anything that has ever been presented to us."[7]

Here then, at a critical moment of historical significance, an opportunity arose for the trustees of the M. D. Anderson Foundation to take a leading role in bringing a medical school to Houston and in the process add an indispensable component to their future medical center. Some thirty years later, Freeman recalled those early meetings and the remarkable timing of it all: "Things were moving forward [plans for the Texas Medical Center] and in our discussions with Dr. Bertner, he emphasized time and again the importance of having in the medical center, in addition to the hospitals, all the components of health education: medicine, dentistry, nursing, and the related professions." The cancer hospital was making progress in its temporary home, and at the time, all indications were that the legislature soon would approve making the

Texas Dental College a part of the University of Texas. Discussions were proceeding about public health and nursing schools, but the future Texas Medical Center still lacked the most critical institution, a medical school. It was at this fortuitous time, then, that Carr Collins and D. K. Martin approached the Anderson Foundation trustees about moving the Baylor University College of Medicine to Houston. "We told the Baylor officials," said Freeman, "that if they were going to leave Dallas—and we weren't encouraging them to do that, we certainly wouldn't take such an institution away from a sister city—but if they were going to leave Dallas anyhow, we would like to have them come to Houston. There were many conferences, and we finally worked out a plan that was adopted."[8]

While Martin went to Houston to confer with Freeman, Collins returned to Dallas and telephoned Bates to arrange for an appointment to meet with him, Horace Wilkins, and John Freeman at Bates's office in Houston. Collins and Martin began this meeting with a complete overview of the events as they transpired in Dallas and the attempt by the Southwestern Medical Foundation to assume the control of the medical school. They told the Anderson trustees that if proper financial support could be offered by the Anderson Foundation and if the trustees pledged that they had no desire to exercise control over the administration of the medical school, they believed they could raise support to move it to Houston. "Because of this Dallas controversy," said Collins, "we were very careful to state all the facts in order to be sure that there could be no misunderstanding with reference to the conditions under which Baylor would move to Houston."[9]

During an interview in 1975, Bates recalled how the meetings with the Baylor trustees unfolded. "It just so happened that our law firm had two clients who were trustees of Baylor University in Waco. When they decided to move their medical school from Dallas, because of its fuss with the medical profession up there, they naturally thought of us. There had been quite a lot of publicity about the Anderson Foundation, the cancer research hospital, and the plans for the new medical center." Bates said that he was representing Martin at the time and had served with Carr Collins's father on the Texas Teachers Colleges Board. He said that Baylor president Pat Neff (a former Texas governor) and trustees Earl Hankamer and Ray Dudley "were great friends of ours."

Bates told them that the Anderson Foundation would not try to induce them to leave Dallas, but if they had definitely made up their minds to leave, they would be welcome in Houston as a part of the new medical center.[10]

After this first meeting with all of the Anderson Foundation trustees, Collins and Martin (Martin stated that Kokernot also attended this meeting) returned to their hotel and telephoned President Neff. They told Neff about the meeting with the Anderson Foundation trustees and suggested that he join them for a second meeting about one week later. During this meeting, Collins observed, "The trustees of the Anderson Foundation had given the subject quite a lot of thought and had reached some definite conclusions with reference to the offer that they would make us." The Baylor representatives said they would need about $3 million in order to relocate the medical college to Houston. The Anderson trustees presented their offer, and a series of meetings ensued to iron out the details.[11]

During the first of many meetings between the trustees of the Anderson Foundation and Baylor, the Anderson trustees stated that since the University of Texas was deeply engaged in plans to locate several university facilities in the new medical center, they would want to discuss any proposed relocation of Baylor to Houston with University of Texas officials. According to Carr Collins: "We suggested to President Neff of Baylor that he confer with President Homer T. Rainey of the University of Texas about the entire matter and, accordingly, President Neff, while en route to Houston for the second interview with the trustees of the Anderson Foundation, went by Austin and spent the night in the home of President Rainey. Through this interview with the president of the University, it was made clear that the University had no objections whatever to the proposed removal of Baylor to Houston." For years, some in Houston had entertained hope that the University of Texas Medical Branch in Galveston could be moved to Houston. But it was clear that this was not to be, and in the end Rainey voiced his approval for the Baylor move.[12]

But the Baylor trustees who had voted in favor of the merger agreement with the Southwestern Medical Foundation remained determined to give that merger a chance to succeed. Kokernot, Collins, Martin, and Neff made it known that they had been talking with the Anderson

Foundation trustees and had an offer. According to Martin, their efforts were "resented by many." But it turned out that the Southwestern Medical Foundation was having financial problems of its own. Then, in an effort to curry support in Dallas, its trustees told the mayor and the Dallas County Commissioners Court that they actually had control of Baylor College of Medicine, despite their insistence to Baylor during the merger talks that this was not their intention. The Southwestern Medical Foundation then signed a contract with the city and Dallas County for the use of Parkland Hospital. The foundation guaranteed that the hospital facilities would be used only by a medical college that was not part of any denominational institution. This contract meant that Baylor College of Medicine would be excluded from the use of Parkland Hospital unless it was willing to acknowledge that it was under the governance of the foundation's administrative committee and that the trustees of Baylor University had ceded all control over it. The Dallas City Council approved the contract on March 10, 1943, subject to confirmation by the Dallas County Commissioners Court. Dallas newspapers broke the story, creating shock and a sense of betrayal at Baylor. This led to much discussion and finally an all-day meeting on April 27, 1943, at which the Baylor trustees voted 16-2 to annul the merger agreement.[13]

Following the cancellation of the agreement, events moved quickly. Baylor trustees now gave serious consideration to the notion of moving the College of Medicine out of Dallas and wondered if the trustees of the Anderson Foundation would, in fact, be interested in having the school in the medical center they were planning for Houston. As Dean Moursund wrote, "The question of the trustees of Baylor University was answered by the trustees of the M. D. Anderson Foundation, after conferences between President Neff, the trustees of the university, and the trustees of the foundation. A proposal was drawn up by the foundation with major stipulations that the foundation would provide the Baylor College of Medicine with an adequate campus site in the medical center and would contribute $1,000,000 for construction of a college building and another $1,000,000, payable $100,000 annually, primarily for research." The proposal of the M. D. Anderson Foundation was submitted to the trustees of Baylor University on May 5, 1943. It was clear, concise, and, at a little more than two pages, directly to the point. In part, the letter stated the following:

After giving consideration on the invitation of the representatives of Baylor University to the removal of the Baylor University School of Medicine and the School of Dentistry from Dallas to Houston, the Trustees of the M. D. Anderson Foundation here submit to you the following proposal, based upon your immediate acceptance and the actual removal of your Medical School and Dental College to the Texas Medical Center in Houston being sponsored by the M. D. Anderson Foundation and others:

1. The M. D. Anderson Foundation will furnish and donate to you an adequate and suitable site of twenty (20) acres in the proposed Texas Medical Center to be used solely as a location for the Baylor Medical School and Dental College and appurtenant activities.

2. The M. D. Anderson Foundation will donate to you One Million Dollars ($1,000,000) for construction of permanent buildings for the Medical School and Dental College on the above mentioned site.

3. The M. D. Anderson Foundation will donate to Baylor University for the use of its Medical School and Dental College for medical research purposes One Hundred Thousand Dollars ($100,000) per annum for a period of ten (10) years beginning with the date of the actual removal of the Medical School and Dental College to Houston; said funds to be used on research projects jointly approved by the Baylor Medical School and the M. D. Anderson Foundation.

4. The M. D. Anderson Foundation has agreed with the University of Texas upon locating and establishing in the Texas Medical Center in Houston the "M. D. Anderson Cancer Research Hospital" as well as the Texas Dental College, if the legislature authorizes the University to take over and operate the Texas Dental College. . . . The Foundation has no desire to circumscribe the work to be done by Baylor but does desire to avoid, as we are sure you do, useless and expensive duplication of efforts.

5. This proposal is made with the definite agreement and understanding that the M. D. Anderson Foundation will have no part in the management and control, directly or indirectly,

of the operations or policies of the Baylor Medical School or Dental College. On the other hand, this proposal is made with the understanding that Baylor will continue its long and well established general policy of admitting students of all faith[s] to its Medical School and Dental College and of selecting its faculty and administrative officials on the basis of scholarship and qualification without regard to a religious faith.

We believe that your acceptance of this proposal would materially assist in developing the Texas Medical Center into one of the great medical educational and research centers in America and in developing Baylor Medical School, already a splendid institution, into one of the foremost medical schools of the country.[14]

Most important, in the view of Dr. Moursund and the Baylor trustees, was the fact that the M. D. Anderson Foundation's proposal clearly stated that the foundation would not attempt to assert control over the medical college and expressed the foundation's desire that the college continue its policies regarding faculty appointments and admission of students. For Moursund, this meant that the M. D. Anderson Foundation recognized that the college had been operated for forty years without sectarianism and that the foundation wanted the college to continue its policies without any interference.[15]

The Baylor trustees formally accepted the offer on May 7, 1943, and on the following day, May 8, 1943, representatives of Baylor and the M. D. Anderson Foundation signed the agreement to move Baylor University College of Medicine and Baylor Dental College to Houston. Some time after this, Baylor decided to keep its dental college in Dallas, since the Texas Dental College already existed in Houston. The Houston Chamber of Commerce quickly raised an additional $500,000 for Baylor. The result, as Moursund wrote years later, was that "never before had the future of the medical college been so well assured as it was in 1943. The provision by the M. D. Anderson Foundation for a site in the medical center in Houston . . . without any interference in the control or operation of the college, gave new life to the school."[16]

The M. D. Anderson Foundation's proposal for Baylor to move its College of Medicine to Houston was remarkable in several ways. On the one hand, it provided the indispensable element that had been missing from its proposed Texas Medical Center, a medical school. In doing so it assured that Baylor University College of Medicine could establish its presence in Houston and have a legitimate opportunity to thrive. Years later, Chancellor Emeritus William T. Butler observed: "It is really a remarkable document, and it is one which was developed by Colonel Bates, John Freeman, and Horace Wilkins, and their negotiations with the Baylor University trustees. It outlined in general terms the core of what is needed to create a research-intensive, educational enterprise: First of all, [it provided] the land. Second, it provided the funding to build the building, and third, funds for research."[17]

During these busy months of 1943, Drs. Bertner and Elliott continued to discuss ideas about how to develop a coordinated medical center with all of the individual institutions working more or less in concert with each other, particularly Baylor and the University of Texas. They quietly developed a plan that they could present at the right time, once Baylor was opened and operating in Houston. Elliott prepared the initial draft, which he then discussed with Bertner. Together they took their plan to John Freeman. Out of this discussion came two ideas that have had a monumental impact in the long-term development of the medical center. First, Freeman stated that he believed the medical center should be independent, not affiliated directly with any university. As Elliott later recalled, Freeman had just returned from a trip east where he had visited several independently organized medical educational centers. He thought that an independently organized medical center would have the best prospects for growth by attracting other health research and educational institutions. "All of us accepted this idea as an excellent one," stated Elliott. Second, one of the continuing questions had been what to name this medical center. Houston Medical Center was one obvious choice, but Freeman realized that for the medical center to succeed in the way its founders had begun to envision, it would need support from beyond the city of Houston. "The answer," said Elliott, "was to be 'The Texas Medical Center.' The name was suggested by John Freeman." In this way, then, the Texas Medical Center was born as an independent institution that would welcome educational and research institutions as well as hospitals and other medical facilities in a way that fostered the growth and success of all.[18]

Immediately after they signed the agreement with the Anderson Foundation, Baylor's administrators began making plans to move the medical school and all of its equipment to Houston. Although the financial status of the college had never been more assured, officials now had to find a suitable building in Houston to house temporarily the medical college and its equipment and laboratories. They also needed to recruit faculty and establish hospital affiliations for clinical instruction. The next twelve months would be a crucial period for the future of Baylor University College of Medicine.[19]

In addition to the necessity of finding a temporary home for the college, Moursund had to do some quick fence-mending with the Houston-area medical community. When plans for Houston's new medical center first began to develop, the Harris County Medical Society (HCMS) had formed a fact-finding committee to assist the Anderson Foundation in securing a medical school that might become part of the new medical center. But the developments that led to Baylor moving to Houston had transpired so quickly that there had been no consultation with any representatives of the city's medical profession and no opportunity for the HCMS committee to have any input at all. Feeling slighted by Baylor, Dr. Judson Taylor, chairman of the HCMS Fact Finding Committee, invited Dr. Moursund to meet with the group to present the facts of what had happened and provide an opportunity for the committee members to ask questions and "clarify some obscure points." Moursund accepted the invitation and met with the committee in Houston on May 14, 1943. Present at the meeting with Moursund were Drs. Judson L. Taylor, E. W. Bertner, Claude C. Cody, Walter A. Coole, Everett L. Goar, E. Freeman Robbins, C. O. Sansing, Moise D. Levy, and John M. Trible, president of HCMS.[20]

As the meeting began, Moursund provided an overview of the issues behind Baylor College of Medicine's move to Houston, including the M. D. Anderson Foundation's offer of support for this endeavor. Dr. Goar then raised a major point of contention with the Houston physicians, saying, "The one significant thing that struck us here in Houston was the fact that the move was planned before the medical profession here could say anything about it." Moursund attempted to mollify this concern, stating, "You must be assured that at no time was there any thought of not wanting the cooperation of the medical profession of

Houston." The Houston physicians asked a number of questions, rang-
ing from their concern about the Baptist Church possibly interfering in
the teaching of medicine to the anticipated cost to the school of educat-
ing students. They expressed their misgivings about attempting such a
major undertaking during the war, because so many doctors who might
join the faculty were now away in military service.[21]

After more discussion between the doctors and Moursund, it began
to appear that the issues that caused the ruffled feelings had been resolved to the satisfaction of all present. Dr. Cody then asked Moursund,
"In what way can the Harris County Medical Society be of aid to you
and Baylor Medical College?" Moursund replied: "If there could be a
committee appointed from the Harris County Medical Society to work
with me in the organization of a faculty and to help in the selection of
a chairman for each of the departments, this would be most helpful."
Cody responded, "In other words, you want a liaison committee from
the Society for a while." Moursund expressed an interest in having a
permanent committee and stressed that the medical school would not
interfere with the administration or the staff of its affiliated hospitals.
One of the major areas of controversy that frequently occurs with the
arrival of a new medical school in a community is known as "town and
gown," in which physicians from medical colleges (gown) often take
over in hospitals with which they are affiliated, displacing the local physicians (town) from their administrative positions and often wreaking
havoc on their medical practices. Moursund's pledge not to interfere in
local hospitals was remarkable in a sense and is likely to have put the
local physicians more at ease as they contemplated Baylor's pending
move to Houston.

A question then arose about the role of the Anderson Foundation
and whether it might be tempted to meddle in the affairs of the medical school. Dr. Bertner, a former president of the HCMS, replied that
"the Anderson Foundation have [sic] nothing to do with the administration of institutions financed by them. They furnish money without
any strings." He noted that the only institution that would carry the
Anderson name was the new cancer hospital. "They consulted with Dr.
Rainey of the University of Texas and Dr. Rainey made no opposition,"
said Bertner. "The Baylor Trustees were so anxious to close the contract with the Anderson Foundation that they simply overlooked the

importance of consulting with the Harris County Medical Society." Dr. Levy then summarized what had transpired during the meeting, saying: "Everything has been covered. The [medical] profession here has the idea that they have received the short end of the deal. Leaving all this aside, the thing had to be created in a rapid manner. The whole thing now resolved itself into whether the Harris County Medical Society can be rounded up to give this their wholehearted co-operation." The meeting ended on a positive note, and the members agreed to meet again and then to propose to the HCMS the idea of creating a liaison committee. Soon thereafter, HCMS president Trible appointed this committee, which comprised seven members: Drs. M. L. Graves (chair), J. A. Kyle, John H. Foster, Frank Barnes, G. H. Spurlock, James Greenwood, and A. Philo Howard, all men over sixty-five years of age and highly esteemed by their colleagues. Graves later stated that the committee and Dr. Moursund held a series of conferences to help with the move. "We are honored to have Baylor Medical College move to Houston," said Graves. "Its future is unlimited and its opportunities unbounded." The committee proved to be a great success, and in a later account HCMS noted: "In a surprisingly short time the transplanted school was functioning smoothly."[22]

Moursund's diplomacy proved successful, and he was able to avert what could have been a disastrous row with Houston's medical community. Now, with the support of Houston-area doctors behind the relocation to Houston, his next order of business was the task of finding a serviceable, temporary new home for the medical school. The responsibility for this fell primarily to the three Baylor trustees who lived in Houston: Ray L. Dudley, whom President Neff named to chair the committee, Earl C. Hankamer, and W. W. West. They had all been classmates at Baylor University years before. Neff also named Alva Bryan and Joe Hale of Waco and Everett Brown of Dallas to the committee. Because the medical school was part of an accelerated program to train doctors for the armed forces, they needed to find a building and arrange for the move so classes for the next term could begin on schedule in Houston on July 12, 1943. They found four possible locations, and Dean Moursund then returned to Houston to look them over. Finally, they decided on the old Sears, Roebuck and Co. building on Buffalo Drive. As Hankamer recalled, they had about thirty days in which to convert the old store and warehouse into a medical school. "We moved right ahead with remodeling, hoping we'd get all the priorities we needed—and stay out of jail," stated Hankamer. Like Dr. Bertner in his efforts to remodel The Oaks sufficiently to open the cancer hospital, Hankamer worried that government officials might refuse permission for the remodeling because of the construction restrictions during the war. "They didn't give us much trouble," said Hankamer. "The country needed doctors. Laboratories had to be installed in places where they formerly had sold men's clothing or run the notions department. Those were pretty strange quarters for a medical school, but they worked out all right, and we were ready for the big move in July. It took fifty van loads to move all the equipment and furniture down from Dallas." In about thirty days Baylor had accomplished an improbable, if not impossible, feat. On July 12, 1943, Baylor University College of Medicine opened in Houston and resumed classes with 131 students.[23]

The *Houston Post* published a special celebratory "Baylor Section" in its Saturday, July 31, 1943, edition. Under the byline "Great Future for College Seen by Dean," Dr. Moursund proclaimed, "Now we will be able to go ahead with our work unhampered by financial worries . . . we will be able to proceed with long planned research and teaching projects." The school had a pledge of $2 million from the M. D. Anderson Foundation, with $1 million set aside for building construction and the other half allocated to support research. The Anderson Foundation also promised a gift of a twenty-acre plot of land adjacent to Hermann Hospital and near the Rice Institute in the area that was under consideration for what was now being referred to as the Texas Medical Center. There was also a pledge from the Houston Chamber of Commerce to sponsor a campaign that would raise $50,000 a year for the next ten years. It is no wonder, then, that Dean Moursund was so optimistic about the medical college's prospects in its new home.[24]

Despite all of this optimism and the promise of land on which a new school would be built after the war ended, however, acquisition of the future home site for the proposed Texas Medical Center was not yet completed. The Anderson Foundation's trustees had been looking for a location that would be suitable for their idealized concept of a medical center. They sought assistance from several people, including Dr. Bertner, who had become the trustees' unofficial medical advisor. Because he

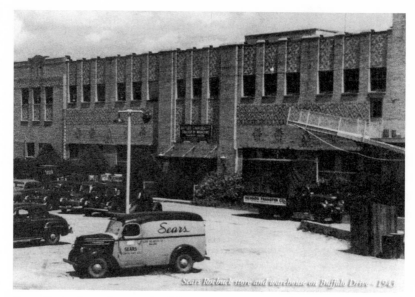

*Sears, Roebuck warehouse on Buffalo Drive, temporary home to Baylor University College of Medicine after the school moved to Houston in 1943. Courtesy of John P. McGovern Historical Collections and Research Center, Texas Medical Center Library.*

had hospital privileges and had served as chief of staff at Hermann Hospital, Bertner was familiar with the large area of land adjacent to the hospital. This was the same land, approximately 134 acres, that Will and Mike Hogg had purchased in 1923 with the idea of offering it to the University of Texas as an inducement to move the Medical Branch from Galveston to Houston. As the story goes, they eventually determined that this idea, whatever its merits in their minds, was unlikely to happen and sold the land to the city of Houston at cost. The land was also flanked on one side by land provided years before by George H. Hermann to be developed into a park, similar to Central Park in New York City, and on the other side by the Rice Institute. The acreage was heavily wooded and swamplike in places, with dense undergrowth. There were a few baseball diamonds in one area, but most of the property was unused. The trustees began negotiations with city officials, and on November 6, 1943, they reached an agreement to purchase that tract of land from the city. But because the site had been intended for park use, city officials and the trustees agreed to put the sale on the ballot to be decided by the people of Houston. Confident that Houstonians would support the proposal, Bates later described his feelings upon reaching the acquisition agreement with the city: "That was a great day. We began to feel that all those dreams of a Texas Medical Center were developing into reality."[25]

On December 14, 1943, in what the *Houston Post* described as "the lightest vote recorded here in many years," Houstonians went to the polls and approved the proposed sale of the 134-acre tract of land to the M. D. Anderson Foundation by a vote of 910 in favor and 41 against. Observers ascribed the light turnout to the lack of any organized opposition to the proposal and also to the cold, rainy weather on that election Tuesday. The favorable vote was the final step to complete the sale of the tract to the Anderson Foundation. The Anderson Foundation would pay the city $318,820 for the tract, $100,000 of which was to be spent for the retirement of the remaining indebtedness on the land and the balance for the purchase of land for twenty-one new public parks. The foundation completed the transaction with the city on April 20, 1944, and purchased a few additional acres, bringing the total to about 140 acres. As Bates recalled, "We thought we had all the land in the world for a medical center, that we'd never need any more." The foundation subsequently provided improvements to the area, which included paving Fannin Street and Holcombe Boulevard, at a cost of an additional $100,000.[26]

Thus, 1943 proved to be one of the most pivotal years, not only for the M. D. Anderson Foundation, but also in the early history of the Texas Medical Center. The Anderson Foundation trustees, William Bates, John Freeman, and Horace Wilkins, were key players in these events in that they were men of integrity, highly respected in the state, able to envision a magnificent medical center for Houston, and willing to make bold decisions in a timely manner when it counted most. Their early support for locating the new state cancer hospital in Houston, coupled with their backing of Frederick Elliott's plan to assimilate the Texas Dental College into the University of Texas, were the first steps in creating a medical center in Houston. Their ability to seize the opportunity when Baylor trustees first approached them about moving the medical school to Houston must be viewed as one of the signal events in making their vision for a medical center into reality. And the acquisition of an undeveloped tract of land that was of suitable size and location on which institutions could construct new buildings all but made their medical center a reality. Realizing that they would need statewide support for this endeavor, early on they named it the Texas Medical Center instead of the Houston Medical Center.

With the opening of the new academic term on July 12, 1943, not only was Baylor University College of Medicine back in business, but each passing day brought greater encouragement to those who had dreamed of creating a medical center in Houston. As important as the arrival of Baylor College of Medicine and the M. D. Anderson Hospital for Cancer Research was for Houston and the Texas Medical Center, none of this likely would have happened without the bold vision and foresight of the trustees of the M. D. Anderson Foundation. As Dr. William T. Butler noted, "I would say that there is absolutely no question that the M. D. Anderson Foundation was critical in bringing Baylor College of Medicine to Houston. This took real foresight. These guys knew what they were doing. They had an image, they had a vision, and we [Baylor] were able to come here and help them realize their dream. But they needed a vehicle to do it and the vehicle was Baylor College of Medicine." A jubilant William Bates later reflected on the support in the Houston business community for the Baylor move to Houston. "As a result of this cooperation and generosity," said Bates, "Houston now possesses the Baylor College of Medicine, one of the great medical schools in the country, as the principal instructional unit in the Texas Medical Center."[27]

The trustees of the M. D. Anderson Foundation had achieved a spectacular success and assembled the initial building blocks required to create a medical center with breathtaking speed for such an endeavor. But the country was still at war, new construction was still prohibited, and not one spade of dirt had been turned for the new medical center. Though much had been accomplished on the way to building the medical center, even greater challenges would arise as soon as the war was over.

# Chapter 7

## "One of the Greatest Medical Centers Ever Developed"

By the first months of 1944, the M. D. Anderson Foundation trustees could list a cancer research hospital, a medical school, a dental college, and a 134-acre tract of land as core components of their planned medical center in Houston. Although many people would have a part in creating the Texas Medical Center during the formative years of 1942–62, undoubtedly it was the collaborative effort of the trustees of the Anderson Foundation along with Drs. E. W. Bertner and Frederick C. Elliott that became the driving force behind the center's early development. In particular, Bertner emerged as both the guiding hand behind the formation of the medical center and the public face in front of it. In fact, while wartime restrictions on construction slowed the physical development of the new medical center, those limitations allowed time for Bertner to work closely with the Anderson trustees and his trusted colleague Elliott in the crucial early stages of planning the medical center.

Bertner's first priority during 1944, however, was preparing the M. D. Anderson cancer hospital to begin serving patients. Although he and his team worked very hard to prepare the old Baker estate, his wife, Julia, was not impressed. "I didn't think that anything could ever come out of it," she recalled years later. "But bless his heart they worked at it so hard." Bertner was a demanding taskmaster and quickly realized that he needed someone who possessed both the professional experience and the fortitude to work under the pressure involved with setting up the new facility. He contacted his former nurse, Anna Hanselman, who had worked with him during the 1920s, and asked her to return to Houston from

California to help organize the new hospital. Bertner had managed to get permission from the government to construct a small clinic building on the estate and wanted Hanselman's help as he prepared it to begin seeing cancer patients. For a time, Hanselman took up residence in the old Baker mansion, where she worked for a year making preparations, gathering supplies, and scrounging for equipment, all of which proved to be a real hardship due to the rationing of most commodities for the war effort. Years later, Hanselman recalled some of the challenges she faced getting the clinic ready. "They were just laying the foundation for the clinic when I got there," said Hanselman. "I had so much to do. You see, you couldn't buy linens and things like that. I spent from about the first of August until the clinic opened making towels and all that we needed for the clinic. I knew everything we'd need because I had worked in Dr. Bertner's office and I had it all ready." One of the final preparatory tasks was for Hanselman to organize, label, and sterilize all of the new instruments in time for the clinic's opening.[1]

Finally, on February 17, 1944, a host of dignitaries, including officials from the University of Texas, the M. D. Anderson Hospital for Cancer Research, and the M. D. Anderson Foundation, held dedication ceremonies for the hospital. Bertner, who was now both chairman of the state cancer committee and acting director of the hospital, presided at the three-hour ceremony. An elated Representative Arthur Cato of Weatherford, who had introduced the legislation to establish the cancer hospital in 1941, exclaimed, "This is the happiest moment of my life!" That evening, at a dedication dinner sponsored by the Houston Chamber of Commerce, Texas governor Coke Stevenson said that the hospital was "a product of men of vision." Bishop Clinton S. Quin opened the dinner program with an invocation, and Francis Marion Law, chairman of the Chamber of Commerce Educational Committee, presided. In his remarks Law paid tribute to Monroe D. Anderson and, looking ahead to the postwar era, also set high expectations for the future Texas Medical Center. "What an inspiration and a challenge Monroe Dunaway Anderson has left to us," he said. "We know that great industrial development is coming to our city; it is pleasing to know that we are not neglecting the humanities. This medical center is to be one of the chief assets not only of Houston and of Texas, but of these United States."[2]

The M. D. Anderson Hospital for Cancer Research officially opened on March 1, 1944, but with only limited services for patients and light research activity. The hospital admitted only needy patients who had no facilities for treatment in their home communities. Thus, Bertner and his team already looked forward to the end of the war, when services could be expanded at the Baker estate and a new building constructed in the Texas Medical Center. In time, more patients began to arrive, and eventually the prevention clinic was converted to provide more room for the patients that were being sent in by the doctors from out of town. "It was gradual," said Hanselman. "I don't think anybody worked harder than Dr. Bertner did to get that Medical Center and Anderson Hospital going."[3]

The Anderson Foundation had hired H. A. Kipp, an engineer who had been involved in developing the area around the Houston Museum of Fine Arts, Hermann Park, and the Houston neighborhoods of Shadyside and Broadacres, to draw up plans for the medical center site. Kipp met frequently with Bertner and accompanied him on several visits to medical centers around the country, eager to see firsthand some of the best practices that could be incorporated for the Texas Medical Center. Julia Bertner also went on many of these exploratory journeys with her husband. "Doctor and I traveled all over this country, looking at different medical centers before he could finally make up his mind about what he wanted to do." She noted that visitors came to Houston from many cities, including New York and Chicago, to share ideas and talk about the medical center. "I tell you, our life was something. I was going from morning 'til night, and so was he, to entertain all of these visiting 'firemen.' We had all of our meetings up there in the Rice Hotel. It kept on right up to the time Doctor died." Bertner and Kipp planned an extensive trip for September, during which they would visit medical centers at Duke University and in New York, Chicago, Philadelphia, Pittsburgh, Washington, DC, and Toronto, all as a means to glean ideas for the layout, construction, and beautification of the Texas Medical Center.[4]

But at midsummer, just a few weeks before the scheduled trip, a challenge reared up that threatened the future of the fledgling medical center, and it arose from a surprising source: the University of Texas. On July 15, 1944, University of Texas president Homer P. Rainey presented a report to the board of regents, a strategic plan for the future of the university, entitled "The Future Development of the University of Texas." In this report

Rainey proposed moving all of the units of the university, including the medical school, dental branch, and the cancer hospital, to the main campus in Austin. This would have meant closing the Medical Branch in Galveston and likely would have killed off or seriously set back the Texas Medical Center in Houston before it ever had a chance to get established. Following his presentation, Rainey asked the board of regents to approve his recommendation. Instead, Judge Dudley Woodward Jr., chairman of the board of regents, referred the report to the board's medical committee. Elliott, dean of the University of Texas Dental Branch in Houston, wrote in his memoir that Rainey's recommendations initiated a "vociferous and drawn out controversy." Woodward appointed a special investigative committee of three members of the board's medical committee, H. H. Weinert, Orville Bullington, and Judge D. F. Strickland, to assess the Rainey report.[5]

During August, while the committee reviewed Rainey's plans for the University of Texas, the Chamber of Commerce's *Houston Magazine* published an article, "Plans for Southwest's Greatest Medical Center Progress," highlighting the Texas Medical Center and the role of the Anderson Foundation trustees in its development. "As a result of the exceptional philanthropy of one man," the article stated, "the efficient administration and wise decision of three able trustees of this vast estate, and the added generosity of a group of Houston business leaders, plans are now under way which are soon to develop . . . the largest and finest medical center in the Southwest." The author observed that it was fortunate for Houston that the Anderson Foundation trustees "decided to make the Texas Medical Center one of the most important and possibly the most favored of all the projects which the M. D. Anderson Foundation will execute." Concluding with what could be described as a combination of gleeful anticipation and civic boosterism, the author reminded readers that although Houston business leaders had long entertained dreams of a medical complex, it was because of "the great generosity of one man and the foresight and civic patriotism of those who now represent him, [that] this dream is being converted into a magnificently planned and well financed reality . . . one of the nation's greatest health and medical centers." But now, it appeared that the fate of that "finest medical center in the Southwest" was left hanging in the balance while the University of Texas considered what to do about Rainey's recommendations and the threat they posed to this dream.[6]

The answer came when the special committee released its findings on September 29, 1944. In view of the fact that the committee members and Homer Rainey had been at loggerheads for several years, it was not completely surprising that their report concluded that all schools of the university should remain in their present locations. Ominously for Rainey, however, the committee stated, "While it seems there are two schools of thought as to whether it is advantageous to have the medical and dental schools on the campus of the Main University, we believe the majority of well-informed opinion is to the effect that it is better not to submerge medical and dental colleges with a Main University. We recommend that it be the policy of the Board of Regents to retain the location of the Medical School in Galveston permanently. We believe that further agitation about removing the Medical School from Galveston should stop, as it is a detriment to the school." Some time later, another special committee of seventy-five citizens affirmed their recommendations.[7]

Homer Rainey had become embroiled in the politics of wartime and in the growing fear that communism was taking root on some of the nation's college campuses. He had taken views that ran counter to most of the university's regents, resulting in a titanic struggle over control of the university and the scope of academic freedom on campus. Stung by yet another rebuke from the board of regents, at a faculty meeting on October 12, 1944, Rainey publicly challenged the regents when he presented a list of sixteen areas of disagreement between himself and the board. The regents reacted quickly: on November 1, 1944, at a meeting at the Rice Hotel in Houston, they voted to fire Rainey. Although some 8,000 students marched to protest his dismissal, the action stood. While one can debate the issues around the Rainey controversy, the end result was that the University of Texas Medical Branch remained in Galveston and the cancer hospital and dental school remained in Houston, fundamental building blocks for the Anderson Foundation's Texas Medical Center.[8]

As the year drew to a close, Bertner gave what became one of the most memorable of his many public addresses regarding the Texas Medical Center. Bertner rarely missed an opportunity to promote the medical center, and he agreed to speak to the Southampton Civic Club at its meeting in December 1944. Elliott also had been invited, and attended the meeting to hear Bertner speak. "His address turned out to be a surprise for all of us and I believe also for Dr. Bertner," said Elliott. "While Dr. Bertner usually followed his notes when making an address, he at times added impromptu remarks. During his address on this day, he hesitated for a moment and then said, 'The Texas Medical Center within a short time will be a development that will exceed $100 million.'" Bertner had mentioned this figure before but not when any reporters were present. According to Elliott, the next morning the Houston newspapers that covered the event carried the story and quoted Bertner's comment about a $100 million medical center for Houston. An article in one of the Houston newspapers caught the eye of an astonished William B. Bates. Elliott recalled that Bertner was on duty at the hospital the next morning and unavailable to comment, so Bates called him instead and asked, "Fred, where is Bill going to get this hundred million dollars? He is not going to get that from us!" Elliott replied, "Colonel Bates, he just got that out of the air—right there at that meeting." The story, quoting Bertner, eventually appeared in newspapers throughout the United States. "Well, Bill and I got tickled by that—we just had more fun about it," said Elliott. "But the idea stuck . . . and that is what built the Medical Center. That one statement made it big, because that hit people and they never forgot it."[9]

By late spring of 1945, the end of the war was finally in sight. Germany surrendered on May 8, 1945, and Japan's emperor Hirohito announced the surrender of Japan on August 15. With the end of World War II, wartime rationing and restrictions on new building construction would soon be lifted. The Anderson Foundation trustees prepared to establish a new entity to which they could hand over the task of managing the Texas Medical Center. John Freeman and other trustees of the Anderson Foundation had in fact already begun discussing plans for a charter to create a new organizational structure for the medical center. Years later, Bates explained their rationale for creating this new entity. "We could see that the medical center was going to move ahead on a very large scale," said Bates. "It needed an organization that would involve a lot of people instead of just the trustees of the Anderson Foundation." Freeman drafted a charter and also sought input from Bertner and Elliott in the process, since both men had given considerable thought to how the medical center should be organized. Finally, on October 8, 1945, the trustees of the Anderson Foundation and representatives from all of the institutions that would initially be in the medical center signed the charter and filed it with the Texas secretary of state, where it was formally recorded on October 20. Texas Medical Center,

Inc., was established as a nonprofit corporation with Anderson Foundation trustees William B. Bates, John H. Freeman, and Horace Wilkins, along with James Anderson, Hines H. Baker, E. W. Bertner, Ray L. Dudley, Frederick C. Elliott, and Bishop Clinton S. Quin as the founding incorporators. At the first meeting of the Texas Medical Center board of trustees, on December 11, 1945, the board elected Bertner president, Freeman vice president, Elliott secretary, and Anderson, who was not related to M. D. Anderson, treasurer. Leland Anderson, a nephew of Monroe, joined the board shortly after it was organized.[10]

During the winter of 1945–46, officials were busy making plans for a dedicatory dinner for the Texas Medical Center, which was to be held on February 28, 1946. Over 600 people attended the banquet, chaired by Ray Dudley, a member of the Texas Medical Center board who also served on the board of Hermann Hospital and as a trustee of Baylor University. Among the thirty people seated at the head table were Anderson Foundation trustees John Freeman, William B. Bates, Horace Wilkins, and Drs. Frederick C. Elliott and E. W. Bertner. The trustees of the M. D. Anderson Foundation invited Leland Anderson to present the deed for the property to the new Texas Medical Center president, Dr. Bertner. In his remarks on behalf of the Anderson Foundation, Leland Anderson said, "It gives me great pleasure to carry out what I know would be the wishes of my late uncle in presenting this deed and promising continued substantial support for the Center." As Ray Dudley introduced Dr. Bertner, he tried to prepare the audience for what was to come. "As you will observe before the next speaker has finished," Dudley said, "he has a boundless vision and an enthusiasm on the subject which brings you here. He has been connected with this enterprise since its inception. He has lived it in his busy days, and he has dreamed of it at night. He will tell you of a wondrous dream, a dream about to come true." Bertner did not disappoint. He called the Texas Medical Center "an economic stride of great importance" and compared it with the Houston Ship Channel as one of the most significant events in Houston's history. "One made Houston's place as a trade center," said Bertner. "The other will make Houston's place as a health center. One brought great commerce; the other will bring great blessings to mankind, and perhaps—who knows—it will bring the answer to the cause, treatment, and cure of cancer. The ship channel brought the captains of industry to our community; the Texas Medical Center will attract the great scientists of the world."[11]

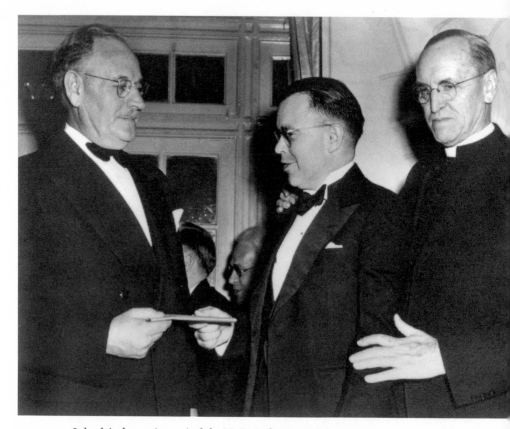

*Leland Anderson (center) of the M. D. Anderson Foundation presenting the deed for the original 142 acres of land to E. W. Bertner (left), president of the Texas Medical Center, February 28, 1946. Also pictured is Bishop Clinton S. Quin. Courtesy of John P. McGovern Historical Collections and Research Center, Texas Medical Center Library.*

Also among the dignitaries who spoke that evening was George A. Hill Jr., chairman of the University of Texas development board. Hill described the Texas Medical Center as being "the fulfillment of the dreams of public-spirited Houstonians, living and dead." He spoke about the key role that the Anderson Foundation had taken in establishing the Texas Medical Center, noting that "the Anderson Foundation, with W. B. Bates, John H. Freeman, and Horace Wilkins as trustees, have laid the framework of the Medical Center by granting funds generously, by wise management and good leadership." This dedication banquet and ceremonies marked a major milestone in the history of the M. D. Anderson Foundation and was a testimony to the important role taken by the trustees in providing not only the initial funds but also the vision and leadership to create the Texas Medical Center.[12]

A few days after the dedicatory banquet, on March 2, 1946, the Houston chapter of the University of Texas alumni organization, the Texas Exes, held its annual banquet in the Rice Hotel ballroom. Some 400 guests again heard George A. Hill Jr., who announced that the M. D. Anderson Foundation was providing an additional $1.5 million contribution to the university's Texas Medical Center program. The new funds were offered in a matching formula, whereby the foundation provided one dollar for every two dollars raised by the University of Texas. The Anderson Foundation previously had given $500,000 toward the erection of permanent buildings for the M. D. Anderson Hospital for Cancer Research and also provided an equal amount for the erection of the dental branch building. In his formal remarks, Dr. Theophilus S. Painter, acting president of the University of Texas, said that he expected the M. D. Anderson Hospital to be "the focal point for cancer research in the state." William B. Bates, a University of Texas alumnus and chairman of the board of trustees of the M. D. Anderson Foundation, noted the significance of the evening, saying: "We are gathered here to launch what is probably the most important single project ever launched by ex-students on behalf of the university." Bates stated that, to him, it was unthinkable that Houston would develop a great medical center and "the University of Texas not be the sparkplug." The foundation's offer spurred a flurry of fund-raising, including additional state funds and a Houston Chamber of Commerce campaign, led by businessman Warren S. Bellows, which raised $1 million for the dental school and cancer hospital.[13]

The Anderson Foundation continued to take a key role in the development of the Texas Medical Center. Years later John Freeman related how the medical center first began to take shape. "Up until late 1945," said Freeman, "we had made commitments to the University of Texas, Baylor, Methodist Hospital, St. Luke's Episcopal Hospital, Shriner's [sic] Hospital for Children, the [medical center] library, and to Hermann Hospital—for expanding their facilities." He noted that every one of the institutions remained autonomous and, apart from the covenants restricting the land to nonprofit use in teaching, research, and medical care, there were no strings attached to the grants from the foundation. The foundation also made financial donations, generally of $500,000, to each of these hospitals for their building fund. "The land was given to them along with an appropriation of money," stated Freeman. "And then that brought in all of the strength of each institution and its backers." Thus, the Anderson Foundation encouraged institutions to come into the medical center by providing them with an appropriate tract of land and with enough seed money to serve as a stimulus to raising additional funds from other supporters. The foundation also invested in infrastructure, including an additional $500,000 for water and sewage mains, grading, paving and lighting of roadways, and surveys to subdivide the land into tracts for the hospitals and other institutions.[14]

Although the Texas Medical Center was now fully under way, its president, Dr. E. W. Bertner, still remained as the interim director of the M. D. Anderson Hospital for Cancer Research. When the war ended in 1945, Bertner strongly encouraged the University of Texas regents to intensify their search for a permanent director of the cancer hospital, knowing that he was about to be named president of the Texas Medical Center. But the regents were having a difficult time finding the right person, someone who would be interested in building a cancer center essentially from scratch. Dudley K. Woodward, chairman of the board of regents, on a visit to the Mayo Clinic in Rochester, Minnesota, expressed his frustration with the lack of results and asked for recommendations. Doctors there told Woodward about an air force physician, Lt. Col. R. Lee Clark, who at that time was stationed at the School of Aviation Medicine, Randolph Field, near San Antonio, Texas. As Clark recalled the story years later, he received a letter from President Painter inviting him to Austin to discuss the position as director of the M. D. Anderson Hospital in Houston. Clark had first heard of the cancer hospital in 1942 and was immediately interested. He recalled that he also found it intriguing that the hospital was the first cancer hospital in this country to be developed as part of a university. "There were a number of people who considered the job," said Clark. "But by early 1946 they still didn't have anybody. Later, whenever I met some of the fellows, they'd say, 'I was offered that job and turned it down. What do you think you're going to do with it in that old house down there?'"[15]

After his first meeting with Painter in February 1946, Clark went through a series of meetings and interviews with the board of regents, Bertner, the Anderson Foundation trustees, and Dr. Alton Ochsner, cofounder of the Ochsner Clinic in New Orleans. Ochsner was a pioneer in cancer research and in 1939 had published one of the first studies linking cigarette smoking and lung cancer. All were highly impressed, and finally Bertner strongly recommended that the regents offer Clark the appointment. He engaged in negotiations over his salary and also about the placement of the cancer hospital within the university's organizational system. Clark insisted that the cancer hospital be an independent entity, not a department of the medical school, and that he be responsible for its budget, institutional program, and building program. He also wanted broader authority over admissions policy and the ability to hire a full-time university staff. These negotiations proved to be crucial for the eventual success of the cancer hospital, showing the wisdom and foresight Clark brought to the job. And this explains, in part, why the M. D. Anderson Cancer Center today remains a separate entity from the University of Texas Health Science Center at Houston. The regents agreed with Clark's requests, and he was formally appointed director of the M. D. Anderson Hospital on August 1, 1946.[16]

One of Clark's first major initiatives as director of the cancer hospital took place the next year. In 1947 several old surplus army barracks at Camp Wallace in Galveston became available. Here again the trustees of the Anderson Foundation took an important role by arranging to purchase twelve buildings from the War Assets Administration for $55,000 and have them moved to Houston, where they were rebuilt next to the Baker mansion. The foundation paid the cost for their relocation, together with the cost of furnishings, equipment, central heating, and air-conditioning, which amounted to nearly $125,000. Warren S. Bellows, president of Bellows Construction Company, arranged for the barracks to be moved to The Oaks and refurbished at cost. Bellows would later serve as a trustee of the Anderson Foundation. According to Bates, the rebuilt barracks "were not too attractive in appearance; but they proved highly serviceable as an admirable pilot plant for the establishment and training of a research staff by Dr. Clark, director of the hospital."[17]

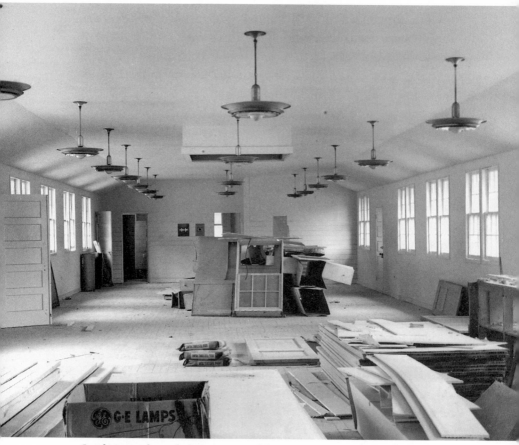

*Surplus army barracks being converted for use at M. D. Anderson Hospital on the old Baker estate, 1947. Courtesy of John P. McGovern Historical Collections and Research Center, Texas Medical Center Library.*

As all of this transpired, Dr. Bertner embraced his leadership role in the Texas Medical Center. This involved countless meetings, planning sessions, and speeches to keep the medical center in the public eye and continue to gain their support. In May 1946 Bertner addressed the Houston Chamber of Commerce. "The combination of Houston's two major developments, the creation of the Texas Medical Center and the designation of this city as an international air gateway, holds promise of making Houston a leader in medicine for Latin American countries," he told his attentive audience. "The populations of Latin America are hungry for medical treatment and research and will look upon the services Houston will have to offer as America's gesture of sound good neighborliness." For months he had been showing architectural drawings of the Texas Medical Center and taking every opportunity to speak in order to gain additional public support. In addition to serving as president of the medical center and maintaining his medical practice, Bertner also continued to function as a leader in the medical profession and in organizations dedicated to fighting cancer. In 1946 he served as head of both professional and lay cancer organizations in the state and in Harris County. In addition, he was vice president of the American Cancer Society at the national level.[18]

Activity continued to increase as more construction began in the Texas Medical Center. During 1947 advocates for a children's hospital formed the Texas Children's Hospital Foundation to develop plans and acquire community support. Several University of Texas institutions received initial approval from the state legislature to build facilities in the Texas Medical Center, including the M. D. Anderson Hospital for Cancer Research and the University of Texas Schools of Dentistry, Public Health, and Geographic Medicine, the Postgraduate Medical School, and the Preceptorial Training Center. Hermann Hospital began construction of a new 400-bed hospital building and a fourteen-story medical office, the Hermann Professional Building. Speculation flew about additional buildings in the medical center that might include facilities for a tuberculosis hospital, a medical library, a blood bank, a marine hospital, several dormitories, four or five fraternity houses, a physicians' residential section, a central power plant, a laundry, shops, and, adjacent to the medical center proper, a 1,000-bed naval hospital. The medical center board formally assigned building sites for new construction to Methodist Hospital, St. Luke's Episcopal Hospital, the University of Texas, and Texas Children's Foundation.[19]

Accordingly, a flurry of construction took place in the Texas Medical Center throughout 1948 and 1949. When a budget shortfall threatened to halt construction on the new Baylor College of Medicine building, Roy and Lillie Cullen made up the difference with an $800,000 donation. When it opened in the Texas Medical Center in 1948, the medical school named the building in honor of the Cullens. The Cullen Building was the first new building in the medical center and was

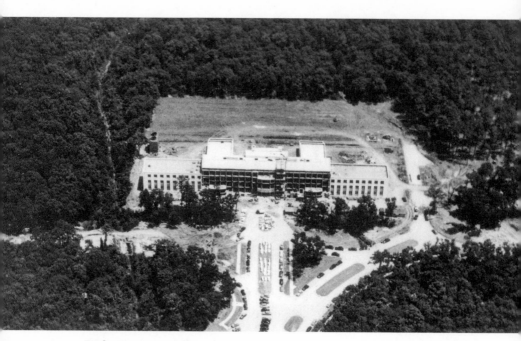

*Baylor University College of Medicine's Cullen Building under construction in the Texas Medical Center, ca. 1946. Courtesy of John P. McGovern Historical Collections and Research Center, Texas Medical Center Library.*

said to be the first air-conditioned structure built in postwar Houston. In 1949 Hermann Hospital opened its new building, and the Hermann Professional Building, located across Fannin Street from the hospital, followed shortly thereafter. The "new building" would in time be named the Robertson Pavilion and was said to be the first air-conditioned major hospital in the United States. Methodist Hospital held groundbreaking ceremonies, the Houston Academy of Medicine moved to the Texas Medical Center, consolidating with the Baylor College of Medicine Library, and the naval hospital was transferred to the Veterans Administration, also becoming the first teaching hospital for Baylor University College of Medicine.[20]

By 1950, the Texas Medical Center was booming with construction and Dr. Bertner continued to wrestle with the challenges posed by the center's rapid development. During the year, the Texas Medical Center board adopted his idea for a fourteen-point policy to guide its efforts and designated a thirteen-acre tract to be the future location for a proposed city-county charity hospital. The board also approved final plans for the M. D. Anderson Hospital for Cancer Research, preliminary plans for the University of Texas School of Dentistry, site development for other University of Texas projects, and plans for the new Arabia Temple Crippled Children's Clinic. The M. D. Anderson Hospital broke ground for its new building, and the boards of St. Luke's Episcopal Hospital and Texas Children's Hospital reached an agreement to construct adjoining buildings and operate under joint administration, an arrangement that would continue for the next thirty-five years.[21]

All of this activity boded well for the future of the Texas Medical Center, but for several months unsettling news had been causing deep concern for its board of directors and for the trustees of the Anderson Foundation. Dr. Bertner had become desperately ill and was engaged in a fight for his life. It all began in 1948, when Bertner developed soreness in the muscles of his left thigh. At first he attributed the problem to a possible muscle strain from climbing a friend's magnolia tree to gather some of the flowers for his wife while on an outing in the country. His medical office partner, Dr. Dudley Y. Oldham, noticed that he was limping when he left the operating room one morning and asked him about it. Bertner explained that he had developed a painful swelling in his left thigh. Oldham encouraged Bertner to take his vacation, which he normally did around late summer, and perhaps the rest would help. Bertner went to Minnesota to do some fishing and to get his annual physical at the Mayo Clinic. The doctors at Mayo did not detect anything serious at that time and advised Bertner to monitor any changes in his thigh. Bertner stayed for a few more days but continued to experience pain. He decided to return to Houston, and two days later, on a Sunday morning, Drs. Lee Clark and Ed Smith examined Bertner and performed a biopsy, after which they determined that Bertner had a rhabdomyosarcoma, a malignant, soft-tissue tumor of the muscles attached to the bones of his thigh. Rhabdomyosarcoma is a rare cancer, and the cause remains unknown even today. Physicians now know that early diagnosis is very important, because it is a very aggressive cancer that spreads quickly. Radiation and/or chemotherapy, in conjunction with surgery, are crucial in treating this vicious malignancy, and chemotherapy is an essential part of the follow-up to prevent further spread of the cancer.[22]

In 1948, however, not much was known about how to treat rhabdo-myosarcoma, and Bertner's doctors had differing opinions on how best to care for their friend. Dr. Clark recommended an aggressive surgery, a hemi-pelvectomy, as the best hope to remove all of the cancer. But the operation would mean the amputation of Bertner's entire left leg and one lateral half of his pelvis on the left side. Neither Dr. Oldham nor Dr. Smith was in favor of this radical surgery, and Bertner immediately rejected the idea, too. The following Sunday, October 3, 1948, Drs. Clark and Smith performed a less severe operation in which they removed the muscle groups in the lateral and upper portions of Bertner's left thigh. He recovered quickly and con-tinued to work with barely any interruption to his schedule.[23]

In the weeks following this procedure Bertner no longer performed surgery, but he continued seeing a few patients in his office. Dr. Mavis P. Kelsey, a friend who also was one of Bertner's physicians during this time, recalled Bertner's indefatigable spirit. "Dr. Bertner was undaunted and exhibited tremendous determination," said Kelsey. "He was soon walking on crutches and going everywhere, including a cocktail party at our house." Bertner focused his efforts mainly on the development of the Texas Medical Center. Within a few months, however, he devel-oped a nagging cough. When a chest X-ray revealed what appeared to be a metastatic lesion in his lung, Bertner went to New Orleans, where his good friend, Dr. Alton Ochsner of the Ochsner Clinic, confirmed the diagnosis. In October 1949, a year after his first operation, Ochsner per-formed a lobectomy on Bertner to remove the cancerous tissue. Once again Bertner rallied, and after a brief convalescence, he was back to work, mainly from his apartment at the Rice Hotel, which gradually be-came his office. Here he dealt with correspondence, held meetings, and reviewed architects' drawings for new buildings in the medical center.[24]

In February 1950 Bertner suffered another setback when he fell in his apartment and fractured his right femur. A biopsy confirmed that the fracture was the result of another malignant bone tumor, an osteo-genic sarcoma or osteosarcoma. There was no choice about treatment, and surgeons amputated his right leg. As winter turned to spring, Bert-ner had more difficulty breathing, and further examination found that the cancer had metastasized, and his lungs were riddled with the dis-ease. Radiation had damaged his left femur, which fractured and had to be pinned. He used a wheelchair and was frequently on oxygen but continued to see visitors from his bed and to write enthusiastically about the Texas Medical Center. A local Buick dealer modified a car to allow easier access and, when duty called and Bertner was up to it, Dallas Johnson, his longtime chauffeur, took him anywhere he wished to go.[25]

On Thursday, June 1, 1950, officials from Methodist Hospital held a cornerstone dedication ceremony for their new building in the Texas Medical Center. The weather that day was bad, but Dallas Johnson helped Bertner to his car and drove him to the ceremony. A special ramp had been constructed so that his car could be pulled up next to the platform. After the ceremony, friends and well-wishers offered greetings to an exhausted Bertner. As Johnson wheeled the Buick onto Fannin Street, Bertner turned to his friend Dudley Oldham and said that he was "finished." A few days later, on June 12, friends and family gathered in his apartment, where Baylor president William R. White conferred upon him an honorary degree of doctor of laws. Among those in the crowded space was Jesse Jones, Bertner's longtime friend and the man who had convinced him to move to Houston almost forty years earlier. Now Jones was a daily visitor to the Bertner home, checking on his friend and offering moral support. Bertner seemed to rally slightly, and on June 19 he and Julia went to their farm in Waller County to enjoy a change of scenery. But after only a couple of days, they returned to their apartment at the Rice Hotel. Despite his obvious suffering, Bertner's spirit never faltered, and he continued to work from his bed. He was on oxygen most of the time, and by mid-July it was clear that he had little time left. Bertner, a true warrior in the fight against cancer, had volunteered himself as a "guinea pig" to try experimental treatments for his cancer. In one final effort, a specialist flew to Houston from the Atomic Energy Commission at Oak Ridge, Tennessee, and gave Bertner a dose of the radioisotope gallium. In his book, *Making Cancer History*, historian James S. Olson wrote of what proved to be a courageous and lasting contribution to medicine by Bertner: "A determination to 'treat to cure' would eventually flower into an M. D. Anderson hallmark, and during the last weeks of his life, Bertner planted the seed. As an institution with a profound research mission, M. D. Anderson had to evolve into a place where patients went to be cured, and the only path to that destination was clinical experimentation." Bertner's willingness to offer himself up for experimental treatment, in hopes of discovering a cure, set a treatment precedent for the M. D. Anderson Cancer Center.

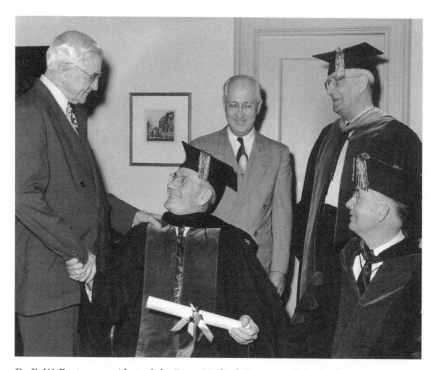

*Dr. E. W. Bertner, president of the Texas Medical Center, receiving an honorary LLD degree from Baylor University, June 12, 1950, just weeks before his death. From left: Jesse H. Jones, publisher of the Houston Chronicle; Bertner (in wheelchair); P. P. Butler, president of the Chamber of Commerce; Dr. Walter H. Moursund, dean of Baylor University College of Medicine; and Dr. W. R. White, president of Baylor University. Courtesy of E. W. and Julia Bertner Family.*

But the radioisotope treatment came too late. Early on July 28, 1950, the man who could rightfully be called the "father of the Texas Medical Center," Dr. E. W. Bertner, died at the age of sixty-one.[26]

Although not unexpected, Bertner's death stunned the medical community. Local newspapers carried the front-page headlines of his passing and printed tributes on their editorial pages. Even before he died, colleagues around the country had recognized Bertner's important role in launching the M. D. Anderson Hospital for Cancer Research and developing the Texas Medical Center. Dr. Cornelius P. Rhoads, one of the world's outstanding scientists in cancer research at Memorial Hospital in New York, wrote to Bertner shortly before he died:

> To see rising a new type of institution, capable, indeed certain,
> of giving leadership to the world, is a most exciting thing . . .
> to know well and to admire deeply the person, yourself, who
> has brought this all about is heartwarming. There can be few
> deeper sources of satisfaction than the creation of new things
> physical, of the mind, and of the spirit. You have done all three
> and more . . . . The structure now at hand is important. That
> to come is unique. But, the soul you have given this unit will
> go on forever, withstand any change and alter substantially the
> course of this country's medical and social progress.[27]

After his death, tributes poured in from all over the country. Bertner's old friend, Dr. Ochsner, spoke to the board of the Texas Medical Center, stating: "We away from Houston think that what you have done here is one of the greatest tributes to far-sighted planning that we have ever seen. The medical profession over the country believes that the Texas Medical Center, as blueprinted during these past four or five years, is the greatest thing that has been started in medicine in fifty years." And John H. Freeman of the M. D. Anderson Foundation, reflecting years later, said, "Consciously or unconsciously, he led us into the concept of the medical center. He visualized the medical center beyond what the rest of us saw and he offered able guidance on technical and professional matters."[28]

In 1971 Dr. William D. Seybold, a distinguished Houston surgeon and a cofounder of the Kelsey-Seybold Clinic, also praised Bertner in his presidential address to the Texas Surgical Society that year. In his eloquent tribute Seybold said, "So ended the life of a man who had fought cancer on every front he knew and with every weapon at his command. His legacy: high spirits, great determination, resourcefulness, imagination, courage, and a magnificent dream to which he gave shape and substance. Ernst William Bertner, the cancer fighter, was cut down by cancer in his sixty-first year. The regiment he led closed its ranks when he fell and moved forward in growing numbers and in increasing strength. Such is his legacy, great is our pride, and large is our debt."[29]

During his professional career, Bertner had become a strong advocate for cancer research. He was steadfast and enthusiastic in his support for the M. D. Anderson Hospital and in his views for the future of the Texas Medical Center. "If we can carry out all that we now have projected," Bertner told a friend, "this will be one of the greatest medical centers ever developed—and I see no reason why we shouldn't."[30]

Bertner's passing was a terrible loss, coming just as the Texas Medical Center was getting under way. But he had planned carefully and created a vision for the medical center that continues, albeit far beyond even his imagination, until today. One of the keys to this continuity is the board of trustees of the M. D. Anderson Foundation. They had bought in fully to Bertner's almost evangelistic vision and would continue to support the Texas Medical Center, in ways great and small, far into the future. But for now it was the Texas Medical Center board of trustees who faced the daunting task of finding a new director. Who could possibly step into the unique role that Bertner had created? It would take nearly two years before the trustees realized that the perfect candidate was before them all the time.

# Chapter 8

## A Building Boom in the Texas Medical Center

Dr. E. W. Bertner's death in July 1950 was a sobering moment in what had been a year of great activity and excitement in the Texas Medical Center. Bertner's leadership shaped the development of the medical center and inspired those with whom he worked. He had been president of the board of trustees and also served as the director. The challenge facing the Texas Medical Center board after his death was to find someone capable of carrying on in his place. The board appointed a search committee to find the right person to serve full-time in the renamed position of executive director of the Texas Medical Center. As the search committee did its work, the dean of the University of Texas School of Dentistry and secretary of the medical center's board, Dr. Frederick C. Elliott, informally stepped into the gap left by Bertner's death and took on many of the director's responsibilities in order to keep things moving forward.[1]

As Bertner's colleagues and friends prepared to carry on without him, planning and construction in the medical center continued unabated. In October 1950 the University of Texas selected the firm of Farnsworth and Chambers to build the new M. D. Anderson Hospital for Cancer Research. Two months later, on December 20, officials and guests gathered as representatives from three women's civic organizations that had actively supported the cancer hospital—the Business and Professional Women's Club, the Texas Department of the American Legion Auxiliary, and the Texas Federation of Women's Clubs— each turned a shovel of dirt, breaking ground for the new building.

Among the dignitaries present were Leland Anderson, vice president of the board of trustees of the Texas Medical Center; William B. Bates and John H. Freeman of the M. D. Anderson Foundation; state senator Searcy Bracewell, representing Governor Allan Shivers; Houston mayor Oscar Holcombe; oilman and philanthropist Hugh Roy Cullen; and a delegation from the University of Texas led by Chancellor James P. Hart, the principal speaker at the ceremonies. Hart expressed the hopes of many that the new hospital one day would be able "to reduce and

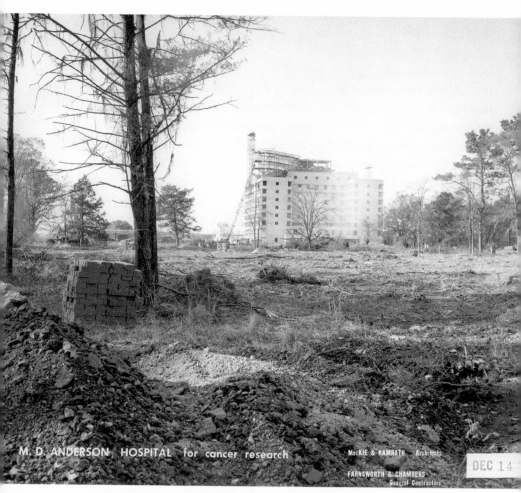

M. D. ANDERSON HOSPITAL for cancer research    MacKIE & KAMRATH    Architects
FARNSWORTH & CHAMBERS    General Contractors    DEC 14

*Construction at the Texas Medical Center, 1950. Courtesy of John P. McGovern Historical Collections and Research Center, Texas Medical Center Library.*

perhaps eventually to end the ravages of one of the most mysterious and dreaded diseases to which the human body is subject."[2]

In a sense, the groundbreaking ceremonies for the cancer hospital marked the end of the Bertner era of the Texas Medical Center. The two institutions to which Ernst Bertner had devoted the last years of his life, the cancer hospital and the medical center, were now well under way. And, as 1950 faded into 1951, both the Texas Medical Center and the M. D. Anderson Foundation began a new phase in their respective histories. The next ten years would bring the first of several periods of extensive expansion and booming construction as new institutions formally joined the medical center. At the same time, the Anderson Foundation continued to provide generous grants to help fund these institutions. In many cases, grants from the Anderson Foundation played a dual, crucial role. First, and obviously, they provided much-needed financial support. But these grants also served an important function as seed money that enabled institutions to seek additional or matching funds from other philanthropic institutions and donors.

During the years 1951–55, construction of new buildings for seven institutions reached completion. When officials from St. Luke's Episcopal Hospital and Texas Children's Hospital held dedication ceremonies at their adjacent sites on February 20, 1951, this event, then, marked the beginning of a new era characterized by booming construction in nearly every corner of the Texas Medical Center. Following these groundbreaking ceremonies, on May 5, the state legislature appropriated $2.4 million for construction of a new University of Texas School of Dentistry that would be located in the Texas Medical Center, near the new M. D. Anderson Cancer Hospital. Shortly after this announcement, on May 17, officials representing Texas Children's Hospital signed a contract with the Tellepsen Construction Company to build their new hospital in the medical center. The following week, on May 23, many of these same officials and other supporters attended the official groundbreaking ceremonies. Construction would begin in mid-July, adding to the seemingly endless movement of bulldozers and dump trucks traversing the landscape.[3]

Later in the year, the Veteran's Administration announced a $3 million addition to the Veteran's Hospital, a neuropsychiatric unit, which also would serve as a teaching facility for students from Baylor

College of Medicine. And, on October 28, 1951, Episcopal bishop Clinton S. Quin, Hugh Roy Cullen, and Reverend Smith of Palmer Memorial Church joined in breaking ground at ceremonies for St. Luke's Episcopal Hospital. This amazing year ended with the opening of the new, nine-story, 300-bed Methodist Hospital in the Texas Medical Center on November 10, 1951. Among the many dignitaries present for the formal dedication were John H. Freeman of the M. D. Anderson Foundation and Leland Anderson, president of the Texas Medical Center. The hospital had already opened some facilities in its basement on September 15 to house the new Speech and Hearing Center. This new center was welcomed as a place where children with speech and hearing difficulties would be treated, regardless of race or financial status; funds for those who could not pay would be provided by individual donors and the Community Chest. Methodist Hospital officially began accepting patients on November 15 with the arrival of sixty-three patients from its original facility on San Jacinto Street.[4]

Construction activity continued at a furious pace into 1952, as even more institutions disclosed development plans or broke ground in the Texas Medical Center. On January 8 the Houston Academy of Medicine announced its intentions to construct a $1.2 million library in the heart of the medical center. The M. D. Anderson Foundation had provided a grant of $300,000 that prompted physicians and other supporters to raise an additional $150,000 toward the building fund. Still short of money to cover the cost of the new library, the academy received a $600,000 donation from Jesse Jones, making it possible for the project to move forward. The library had been one of Dr. Bertner's highest priorities for the new medical center, and it was fitting that Jones, his longtime friend, would help ensure the building's construction. Bertner viewed the library as an important component, along with a medical school, to making the Texas Medical Center one of the nation's leading medical training and research centers. The library would be housed in a four-story structure located on a 3.3-acre tract of land in front of Baylor University College of Medicine and adjacent to Hermann Hospital. Capable of holding some 140,000 books, it would also have an auditorium, meeting rooms, and administrative offices for the Texas Medical Center.[5]

A few weeks after the library's announcement, on February 16,

1952, seven-year-old Geneva Ann Wright and three other children, patients of the Arabia Temple Shrine Crippled Children's Clinic, helped set the cornerstone for the new $1 million clinic building. Since 1949, Hermann Hospital had provided space for the clinic, and soon it would have its own home. John H. Freeman, the keynote speaker, stressed the importance of the new facility, saying, "In this clinic, children are treated without cost and without any distinction as to color or creed or race." It is interesting to note that during a time of state-mandated racial segregation, many leaders in the Texas Medical Center's institutions, including the trustees of the M. D. Anderson Foundation, quietly worked to ensure better medical treatment options for the city's African American population.

Later in the year, on May 3, a beautiful spring day in Houston, officials and invited dignitaries held groundbreaking ceremonies for the dental school's new building. The Anderson Foundation had taken a decisive role in financing construction of the building by providing grants totaling $1.25 million, one of the largest gifts ever made to a dental school up to that time. More than 500 people attended the ceremonies, including Chancellor Hart of the University of Texas; Mayor Oscar Holcombe; Senator Searcy Bracewell; John Freeman, vice president of the Anderson Foundation; and Dr. Marcus Murphy, president of the Houston District Dental Society. Chancellor Hart and Dean Elliott both expressed their profound appreciation to the Anderson Foundation, whose support, along with $2.4 million appropriated by the state, made the new building possible.[6]

Construction at the Texas Medical Center continued through the summer, with the rumbling sounds of massive bulldozers, earthmovers, and dump trucks reverberating over the landscape and huge cranes bobbing and weaving around each other, all engaged in creating new homes for institutions dedicated to the healing arts. While the grounds of the medical center buzzed with activity, behind the closed doors of their offices in the Hermann Professional Building the medical center's trustees were having no success in finding a successor to Dr. Bertner. Two years had passed since Bertner's death, and still there was no permanent director. Frederick Elliott, as secretary of the board of trustees, had been serving as an unofficial interim director. During his years as dean of the Texas Dental College and now as vice president and dean of the University of Texas School of Dentistry, Elliott had proved to be a very capable executive in addition to being known as an innovative educator. But in their enthusiasm to find the perfect replacement for Bertner, the medical center's trustees had overlooked the talented dental professor and administrator in their midst. Years later, Elliott recalled the day in September 1952 when he received a phone call from Hines Baker, one of the members of the search committee. Baker told Elliott that the committee had been searching for some time for a candidate who could meet the requirements they had determined were necessary in a successful executive director. "I have that man," Baker told Elliott. Elliott waited patiently to hear whom Baker wanted to nominate for the position. "I don't know why I had not thought of this before," said Baker, "but the thought just struck me this morning that you are the man to take this place." Elliott was stunned. He had not been seeking this appointment and was in fact looking forward to continuing as dean of the dental school when it moved into the new building, just now under construction. But Baker told him that the medical center had been too long without a leader, that Elliott in fact had been doing that job already and doing it well. He assured Elliott that in the medical center's offices, he would be physically close to the new dental school and able to maintain his ties to that institution. Baker then asked for Elliott's approval to discuss the idea with the other trustees. While Baker met with them, Elliott held confidential discussions of his own with several of the dental school faculty, staff, and with Chancellor Hart, all of whom expressed their disappointment at the prospect of losing the man who had saved the old Texas Dental College and provided the leadership to bring it into the University of Texas System. He worried over the issue in long discussions with his wife, Ann. "After considerable time and many more discussions with those at the dental school," said Elliott, "I made the decision that if I were offered the position as director of the Medical Center, I would accept."[7]

Within a few days, medical center trustee James Anderson scheduled a meeting with Elliott to inform him that the board had agreed to appoint him as the new executive director of the Texas Medical Center. As Elliott later stated, "I was to become the new head of the Texas Medical Center—a great surprise to the profession, to the people of Houston, and of the state. To them, I had become 'Mr. Dental School.'" As Elliott prepared to assume his new leadership role, the University of Texas began a search for his successor as dean of the dental school. Elliott had recommended three members of the faculty that he thought had the talent and qualifications to serve. The university chose one of those candidates, Dr. John V. Olson, as the new dean of the dental school. On November 1, 1952, Frederick C. Elliott formally took his place as the new executive director of the Texas Medical Center.[8]

Although Elliott no longer served as dean of his beloved dental school, it was fitting and appropriate that he now was called to lead the burgeoning Texas Medical Center. Like his friend E. W. Bertner, Elliott had long dreamed of some sort of medical center for Houston. In many ways the opposite of the charismatic Bertner, he was a self-effacing man who preferred to work behind the scenes, but he was not averse to speaking publicly on behalf of the two institutions about which he cared most, the dental school and the Texas Medical Center. During Elliott's tenure as executive director of the medical center, he skillfully led that institution through a phenomenal period of massive construction projects; all the more remarkable during an era in which a bitter dispute over a city-county public hospital threatened to overshadow all of the "good works" taking place on the campus.

Frederick C. "Fred" Elliott was born in Pittsburg, Kansas, on October 23, 1893. During his childhood years he survived polio and the loss of his mother, who died when he was just four years old. He and his brother began helping their father in his drugstore, and by the time Elliott was seventeen, he had passed the pharmacy board exam. After a few years of attempting to run his own drugstore, Elliott enrolled in the Kansas City Dental College, where he graduated in 1918. He accepted a faculty appointment at the school and discovered his love for teaching. Later in the year, tragedy struck, when both his young wife and their premature baby died, victims of the global flu pandemic. Ten years later Elliott remarried and moved to Memphis, where he was appointed to the faculty of the University of Tennessee College of Dentistry. In 1932 Elliott and his wife moved to Houston, where he became the city's highest-level health educator when he took over as dean of the struggling Texas Dental College. During the next decade Elliott restored both its finances and reputation, making it an attractive prospect to assimilate into the University of Texas System and become one of the first institutions in the Texas Medical Center. The University of Texas took over the college in 1943, when it became the School of Dentistry (often referred to as the Dental Branch at Houston), with Elliott remaining as dean. Three years later he was elevated to a vice presidency of the University of Texas while retaining the deanship.[9]

During the 1930s, Elliott developed a passion for improving public health in Houston and served on the boards of several agencies, including the Red Cross, the Texas State Board of Health, and the Houston Board of Health (of which he was president, 1938–41); he was also a member of the executive committee of the Harris County chapter of the National Foundation for Infantile Paralysis and the chairman of the Houston Chamber of Commerce Health Committee. Elliott also became acquainted with many influential community and political leaders through his work on these local and state organizations, among whom were Col. William B. Bates and Dr. E. W. Bertner. After a speaking engagement in Pittsburgh, Pennsylvania, in 1938, Elliott visited the University of Pittsburgh campus, where he was inspired by the new, forty-two-story Cathedral of Learning. Elliott determined that a similar structure in Houston would be perfect to house a medical education and hospital complex. Subsequently, an architecture student from the Rice Institute, in exchange for badly needed dental care, created a preliminary design that Elliott named the Memorial Center for Health Education. The blueprint called for a medical school as well as schools of dentistry, pharmacy, and nursing to be situated in the lower part of the building, occupying approximately six stories. The upper floors would hold a hospital, located on the top, where it could best catch the cool breezes for patient comfort during a time before air-conditioning in the city. Elliott had a model constructed, and then his dental students made miniature versions out of dental plaster that were used to publicize his idea. For the next three years, until the State of Texas and the Anderson Foundation created a cancer hospital in Houston, Fred Elliott campaigned as one of the leading advocates for a comprehensive medical education center in the city. His longtime interest in public health and his position as the leader of the only higher-level health education institution in the city, the Texas Dental College, ultimately led to his role as one of the founders of the Texas Medical Center. Elliott's experience as both administrator and educator, his expertise in the field of public health, and years of advocacy for a medical center made him the ideal choice to succeed Bertner and lead the Texas Medical Center during one of the most important eras in its history.[10]

Working from early morning until late at night, Frederick Elliott embraced his new role as head of the Texas Medical Center. He held a series of meetings with administrators of the institutions in the medical center, with physicians, and with various boards of trustees, to open lines of communication, ascertain their concerns, and seek recommendations. Elliott was most effective in these behind-the-scenes situations and proved to be the steady hand that could steer the medical center through the tumultuous days that lay ahead. The days passed quickly, and by the end of November 1952 he had received word that the M. D. Anderson Foundation was about to provide an additional $1.2 million grant to the M. D. Anderson cancer hospital for the construction of the west nursing wing, which had been deleted from the original plans due to budget constraints. One floor of the wing would be named the Bertner Memorial Wing in honor of the hospital's first director. Once again, the foundation had a larger impact than the amount of its gift because the donation encouraged others to support the new wing through donations to provide the furnishings and equipment.[11]

Although this announcement was heartening news for Elliott, the first weeks of his tenure were filled with both highs and lows. Early in 1953 events took a more positive turn when the trustees of the Texas Medical Center voted to elect W. Leland Anderson president of the board. Anderson had been deeply involved in the Texas Medical Center almost from its inception, and his steady leadership would serve the board well for the next twenty-three years, until 1976. In addition to this good news, late spring also brought the opening of Texas Children's Hospital. On May 15, 1953, Leopold Meyer, J. S. Abercrombie, and many others were present as their long campaign for the hospital finally came to fruition. Dr. Stanley Olson, who succeeded Walter Moursund as dean of Baylor University College of Medicine, served as the principal speaker.

The year passed quickly, but as summer turned to fall, sorrow again visited the Texas Medical Center and the board of trustees of the M. D. Anderson Foundation. Horace M. Wilkins, the man who had succeeded Monroe Anderson on the foundation's board of trustees, developed a sudden illness and was admitted to Hermann Hospital in critical condition. He died at the hospital on Sunday evening, September 13, 1953, at age sixty-eight. In addition to having served on the Anderson Foundation board of trustees since 1940, Wilkins was one of the original founders of the Texas Medical Center. He also was a trustee of Shriners Hospital for Children and had served as the treasurer of the Texas Episcopal Diocese for many years. Bishop Clinton S. Quin conducted funeral services on Monday, September 14, at the George H. Lewis & Sons Funeral Home. Following the service, Wilkins's remains were sent to Hopkinsville, Kentucky, his wife's hometown, for burial. Wilkins was held in high esteem in the Houston business community and recognized for his banking expertise and his selfless service on behalf of many charitable institutions. Years later, William B. Bates paid tribute to Wilkins, noting, "He was a very wise trustee, with farsighted vision, sound judgment and discretion, and deserves a full share of credit for all worthwhile accomplishments and contributions of the foundation during his time as a trustee."[12]

The following year, 1954, proved to be an active year at the medical center as many institutions moved into their newly completed buildings. Because of all this activity, on February 14, the *Houston Chronicle* published several special articles about the M. D. Anderson Foundation. The articles reported that the foundation had awarded some $14 million in grants since its inception and that the corpus had grown to approximately $24 million. Bates modestly attributed the gain to inflation, but the paper stated, "Local financial circles credit the major part due to sagacious management and administration" of the foundation. The trustees had authorized the sale of some of the foundation's shares of Anderson, Clayton stock, which brought in $3 million. They also sold the Seaport Oil Company, part of Monroe Anderson's holdings, for a 100 percent profit. During the 1940s, the foundation had acquired the Shell Building and later sold it for a profit of some $500,000. The trustees managed an investment portfolio with stocks and bonds that returned, on average, about 5 percent, or $1.2 million on an annual basis. In addition to providing grants to worthy institutions, the foundation made available approximately $1.5 million in real estate loans to local churches, including African American churches, which found it particularly difficult to secure loans during the time of Jim Crow

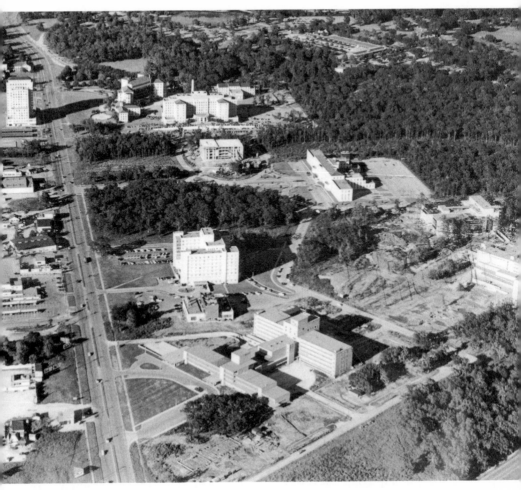

*Texas Medical Center, aerial view, 1953. Courtesy of John P. McGovern Historical Collections and Research Center, Texas Medical Center Library.*

segregation. Bates noted, "We believed that when we made a church loan, we not only had an income investment, but also we were aiding in development of the social and spiritual life of the community." William Bates and John Freeman had been running the foundation since Horace Wilkins's death months earlier. But a few days after the *Houston Chronicle* articles, they announced that Warren S. Bellows would fill the vacant seat on the board of trustees. Bellows owned Bellows Construction Company and had been long involved as a civic leader, supporter of the cancer hospital, and patron of the medical center. He would serve on the board until 1967.[13]

The following week, on February 26, 1954, movers began hauling equipment from the original location of the M. D. Anderson Hospital for Cancer Research, the old Baker estate, to the new 320,000-square-foot, Georgia pink marble building in the Texas Medical Center. Fittingly, a few weeks later, on March 19, just as winter turned to spring, hospital staff tenderly loaded the forty-six cancer patients into a caravan of ambulances for the transfer to the new building. Since first opening ten years earlier, the M. D. Anderson Hospital for Cancer Research had treated over 13,000 patients. This day marked the beginning of a new phase in the history of the hospital and also a consequent new era in the history of cancer research. It was also a monumental day for the Texas Medical Center, since it was the founding of this hospital in 1941 that had been the catalyst for creating the medical center. The beautiful new building consisted of four sections that included two six-story wings for patient rooms (with partial seventh-story offices and rooftop garden), a five-story medical services wing, and a five-story wing to house research laboratories. A few weeks later Dr. Lee Clark unveiled a portrait of Monroe D. Anderson in the hospital named in his honor. It was during this time, the spring of 1954, that the hospital began using a new name, the University of Texas M. D. Anderson Hospital and Tumor Institute. The board of regents formally adopted this name on May 13, 1955.[14]

The cancer hospital was formally dedicated in the fall as part of a three-day scientific conference that included symposia on cancer research for basic scientists, panel discussions and clinical conferences for physicians, and a series of general-interest presentations, all of which culminated in the official dedication ceremonies on Saturday, October 23, 1954. Tom Sealy, chairman of the board of regents, presided over the ceremonies, which included Arthur Cato, who had introduced the bill to create a cancer hospital in 1941. Also present were a host of dignitaries: Governor Allan Shivers, who gave the keynote address; Dr. Logan Wilson, president of the university, who read congratulatory messages from President Dwight D. Eisenhower and from Oveta Culp Hobby, the secretary of health, education, and welfare; US senator Price Daniel; Harris County judge Bob Casey; Mayor Roy Hofheinz; John Freeman, president of the board of the M. D. Anderson Foundation; and many others, including a very special guest, Julia Bertner.[15]

Now that the cancer hospital was formally opened, Elliott continued to lead the fast-growing development of the medical center. In June he and his administrative staff moved the medical center's administrative offices from the Hermann Professional Building to the fourth floor of the new Texas Medical Center Library in the Jesse H. Jones Library Building. On July 16, the Doctor's Club opened its facility on the third floor of the building, and soon trucks began bringing boxes filled with books, journals, and equipment from other libraries in the medical center. Finally, on September 10, officials formally opened the new library. Many prominent citizens of Houston and elsewhere were present. Dr. Chauncey Leake, the executive vice president of the University of Texas Medical Branch at Galveston, served as the keynote speaker. Among the many dignitaries present was Jesse Jones, who received a plaque in appreciation for his donation, which had enabled construction of the new building.[16]

On October 6 officials held dedication ceremonies for the recently opened St. Luke's Episcopal Hospital. The new hospital, with 300 beds and 218 physicians, was a source of pride for Houstonians and particularly for Episcopalians. Wright Morrow, president of the hospital's board of trustees, presided over the ceremonies, and Bishop Quin, who had been deeply involved with the medical center from its inception, formally dedicated the hospital. Dr. Frank R. Bradley, president of the American Hospital Association, was the principal speaker. The Episcopal Diocese of Texas had launched a fund-raising drive to build the hospital in 1946. During their long fund-raising campaign, Hugh Roy Cullen donated $1 million for construction of the hospital, an amount similar to what he also provided to Methodist Hospital, Memorial Hospital, and the Catholic hospital, St. Joseph's. Hugh Roy Cullen and his wife, Lillie, were stalwarts in their support for many institutions of the Texas Medical Center, a fact noted with much appreciation by William Bates on several occasions. City officials recognized this generosity too and declared November 29, 1954, "Hugh Roy Cullen Day" in Houston.[17]

The furious pace of construction that characterized the first eight years of the Texas Medical Center slowed somewhat during the late 1950s. What happened during these years, however, ultimately drove the next period of construction and expansion. The hospitals in the medical center soon became overcrowded due to the steady increase in the number of patients treated. The late 1950s, then, saw administrators hiring architects and seeking more financial support as they struggled to find room to expand their facilities to handle the growing demand. During this time physicians also began to grasp the significance of what was happening in the Texas Medical Center and became increasingly aware of its growing prominence. On July 18, 1955, the Postgraduate Medical Assembly of South Texas recognized the role of the M. D. Anderson Foundation and trustees William B. Bates and John H. Freeman at a luncheon held in their honor. The assembly presented plaques to Bates and Freeman for their "unselfish devotion to humanity and outstanding contributions to medicine and surgery." And later in the year, on December 2, 1955, Elliott enjoyed the satisfaction of attending the dedication of the new University of Texas Dental Branch building in the Texas Medical Center. The school had opened on June 6, when the staff moved their equipment from the old School of Dentistry on the corner of Fannin and Blodgett Streets to the school's new five-story, 198,000-square-foot home. The dedication included a testimonial dinner attended by Dr. Logan Wilson and the entire University of Texas board of regents, who honored Elliott for his years of advocacy for the new building.[18]

During the next year, the M. D. Anderson Foundation continued to support the Texas Medical Center and its growing number of institutions. On May 9, 1956, officials gathered to dedicate the new Institute of Religion, the first such institute in the United States to be located in a medical center and the first devoted to medical ethics. The M. D. Anderson Foundation had provided a grant to the nondenominational institute, which was designed to "challenge and explore issues of faith, health, and healing" and to provide training for theological students to serve as hospital chaplains. The institute began operations a few months earlier in temporary facilities in the Jesse H. Jones Library Building. It would take another four years for the institute to raise the needed funds and begin construction of its own building.[19]

Later in May officials at Methodist Hospital announced that planning was under way for its first building expansion to accommodate the large number of patients seeking treatment at the hospital. A few weeks later, on June 26, the University of Texas board of regents approved architectural plans for a $980,000, 19,500-square-foot expansion of the M. D. Anderson Hospital and Tumor Institute. Funds would be used to extend the loading dock and create storage space for records, build a new super-voltage room to house a second cobalt-60 treatment unit, and enclose the entire seventh floor open-deck area, which would be converted for the administrative offices, most of which were located on the first floor. The vacated first-floor space would be used to expand the outpatient clinic, which had become dangerously overcrowded at times due to a steady influx of new patients, many of whom now were coming from all over the United States as the hospital's reputation continued to grow. As plans for this new construction were unveiled, the M. D. Anderson Foundation announced that it was awarding a $500,000 grant to the recently established University of Texas University Cancer Foundation, to be paid in equal amounts of $100,000 over a five-year period, thus assuring the future of the foundation.[20]

Near the end of the year, on November 20, 1956, William Bates, then serving as vice president of the M. D. Anderson Foundation, addressed the first meeting of the Texas Gulf Coast Historical Association. His written remarks, entitled "History and Development of the Texas Medical Center," became one of the first written accounts of the history of the medical center and the central role of the M. D. Anderson Foundation in creating it. In his presentation Bates provided a brief biography of Monroe D. Anderson, an overview of the development of the medical center up to 1956, and a summary of the grants the M. D. Anderson Foundation had given to institutions in the medical center apart from what it had provided for the M. D. Anderson Hospital and Tumor Institute. The list included $500,000 each to Arabia Temple Crippled Children's Hospital, the new Hermann Hospital, Methodist Hospital, and St. Luke's Episcopal Hospital. The foundation had also provided grants of $400,000 to Texas Children's Hospital, $350,000 toward the cost of the medical library building, and over $60,000 for the library to acquire books and research material for its collections in order to "build up for the Center one of the great medical research libraries of the world." Bates also acknowledged the importance of contributions from others who helped build the medical center, including Lillie and Hugh Roy Cullen, who by then had given some $9.6 million to

Houston's medical institutions; Lillie and James S. Abercrombie, whom he called "the principal benefactors of the Texas Children's Hospital"; and Mary Gibbs and Jesse H. Jones, who had donated $600,000 toward the new library building.

Bates also briefly summarized some of the other activities of the M. D. Anderson Foundation during its first twenty years. The foundation initiated the acquisition of 2,400 acres of land near Conroe, Texas, for what later became Camp Strake of the Sam Houston Council of Boy Scouts, and later provided $25,000 for camping and outdoor equipment. The foundation provided $300,000 to help the Rice Institute purchase a half-interest in the Rincon Oil Field, which had reached an estimated net worth of $30 million by 1956. The foundation also acquired ninety acres of land adjacent to the University of Houston and donated it as an adjunct to the campus. In addition to this grant, the foundation provided $1.5 million to construct the M. D. Anderson Memorial Library on the University of Houston campus. The foundation had made many grants to other hospitals, schools, and many other institutions and organizations, such as the YMCA. Bates explained how the trustees had sold Monroe Anderson's interest in the Seaport Oil Company and some $11 million in Anderson, Clayton & Company stocks and then invested those funds to the benefit of the foundation. In all, Bates stated that, by November 1956, the M. D. Anderson Foundation had made grants of over $18 million and had built up the corpus of the foundation to over $25 million. "It is the policy of the Trustees," said Bates, "to make all donations out of income and preserve the corpus as a perpetual fund that the income down through the ages may be used for the promotion of health, education, and the general welfare of the community."[21]

Although there was a bit of a lull in construction activity during the next two years, 1957–58, two institutions announced plans to begin major construction. On June 6, 1957, officials at Methodist Hospital announced that its board had approved plans for a $7.5 million expansion. And on July 9 Anderson, Clayton & Company executive Lamar Fleming Jr., who also served as president of the Texas Institute for Rehabilitation and Research announced that it now had sufficient funds to build a hospital for the institute, which had been operating in temporary facilities. And in February 1958 the medical center allocated a tract of ground near Baylor University College of Medicine for the new sixty-bed Houston State Psychiatric Institute for Research and Training.[22]

During the next summer, on July 24, 1958, the Texas Medical Center took a tentative step into the future when it opened a helipad for an air ambulance service, just south of St. Luke's Episcopal Hospital. As part of the ceremonies, Houston mayor Louis Cutrer arrived on the landing pad by helicopter and was greeted by Leland Anderson, president of the medical center, and a number of hospital administrators. The new service, operated by Airlift Inc., would be available to bring out-of-town emergency patients who arrived by airplane from the airport to the medical center. It also would be ready to transport accident victims quickly to the medical center's hospitals, saving precious time and lives. Surprisingly, this pioneering air ambulance program lasted only a few months. No one requested the helicopter service, and it soon went out of business, with the landing pad converted to parking spaces. Fifteen years later, in 1973, businessman John S. Dunn donated funds to establish the John S. Dunn Helistop at Hermann Hospital. This subsequently led Dr. James "Red" Duke to establish the Memorial Hermann Life Flight helicopter ambulance service in 1976.[23]

One of the year's last major events in the medical center took place one week after the opening of the helipad, on July 31, when officials held groundbreaking ceremonies for the Speech and Hearing Center. The M. D. Anderson Foundation had contributed $150,000 for the new facility. Drs. Charles Dickson and Herbert Harris, along with J. S. Cullinan II and insurance magnate Gus Wortham, formed a committee to raise the remaining funds to construct the building. The Cullinan family and Gus Wortham were successful in business and had generously dedicated much of their fortunes to such philanthropic pursuits.

The pace of construction in the Texas Medical Center picked up in 1959 and continued into the early 1960s. In January 1959 officials from the Texas Medical Center and Baylor University College of Medicine announced a new, cooperative endeavor with the formation of the Joint Administrative Committee of the Texas Medical Center and Baylor University College of Medicine. Attorney Leon Jaworski was appointed to chair this committee, formed for the purpose of developing a closer working relationship between the two institutions in order to construct three badly needed new buildings for the medical school. Jaworski had been a rising star since joining Fulbright, Crooker, & Freeman in 1931 and was a good choice to chair this committee. Born September 19, 1905, in Waco, Texas, Jaworski was a graduate of Baylor Law School and later earned a master's degree at George Washington University Law School. In 1925 he became the youngest person ever admitted to the Texas Bar. During World War II, he served in the Judge Advocate General's Corps and was appointed chief of the trial section of the war crimes branch, which conducted over 500 trials in Europe. After the war Jaworski returned to the firm, then known as Fulbright, Crooker, Freeman & Bates. He and William B. Bates are credited with building the firm's oil and gas practice into what would become a major global energy law practice. Jaworski's hard work led to him becoming a named partner in 1954, when the firm changed its name to Fulbright, Crooker, Freeman, Bates & Jaworski.[24]

Just before the committee formed, administrators at Baylor University College of Medicine learned that if they could raise half of the cost for the new buildings, they might be entitled to a matching grant from the Department of Health, Education, and Welfare. However, the school's Baptist administrators in Waco had a strict policy regarding separation of church and state that prohibited seeking funds from the federal government. In this instance, the Texas Medical Center's board of trustees agreed to act on behalf of the College of Medicine and take the lead in raising funds and managing the building program. The M. D. Anderson Foundation gave $1 million to the Texas Medical Center to fund what would be called the Anderson Basic Research Building. Houston Endowment, established by Jesse H. and Mary Gibbs Jones in 1937, provided $1 million for the Jesse H. Jones Clinical Research Building, and individuals from Houston's Jewish community raised $450,000 toward construction of the Jewish Institute for Medical Research. These funds, all given to the Texas Medical Center, enabled the medical center's board of trustees to file the request for the federal grant. The Joint Administrative Committee supervised all planning and construction of the buildings, while the medical school's dean, Dr. Stanley Olson, and the faculty all had input in the planning process. Thus, it was the Texas Medical Center, and not Baylor University, that applied for the federal matching funds. On March 12, 1959, the Texas Medical Center held a dinner to celebrate its anniversary and to announce the ongoing fund-raising

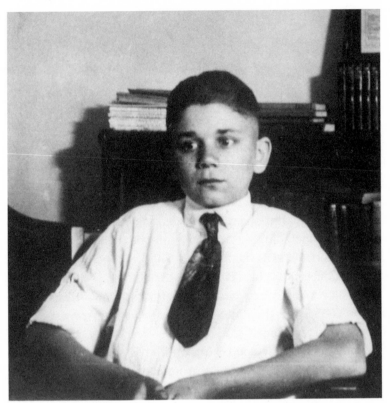

*Leon Jaworski as a youth. Courtesy of Fulbright & Jaworski LLP.*

program for the new Baylor buildings. In all, some $25 million in new construction was either in the planning stage or actually under way in the Texas Medical Center. When added to the $80 million in buildings already constructed, the Texas Medical Center was about to reach the $100 million figure that Dr. E. W. Bertner had spoken about so enthusiastically fifteen years earlier. In the meantime, fund-raising continued for the three research buildings that were to be constructed at Baylor College of Medicine. Near the end of the year, on November 6, officials learned that the Texas Medical Center would receive a $2.4 million federal grant that would match the amount already raised on behalf of the College of Medicine buildings. Once construction of the new buildings was completed, the Joint Administrative Committee disbanded.[25]

Early in 1960, on February 19, the M. D. Anderson Foundation announced a grant of $500,000 to St. Joseph's Hospital to enlarge patient care facilities. Although the hospital was not part of the Texas Medical Center, it served a vital need at its location downtown and also provided opportunities for teaching and research for Baylor University College of Medicine, the University of Texas Dental Branch, and the Postgraduate School of Medicine.[26]

In May the Anderson Foundation released an annual report showing that the foundation's corpus had grown to some $28,550,000 and that over the years the foundation had distributed grants totaling $23,069,103, with over $9 million going directly to the Texas Medical Center and its institutions. The foundation also continued to support universities, including the Rice Institute, the University of Houston, the University of Texas, Texas A&M College, St. Thomas University, and Harding College in Searcy, Arkansas. In addition, grants were also given to smaller colleges, to programs for other activities in the city of Houston, to the YMCA, the Boy Scouts, the Salvation Army, and to a variety of worthy programs.[27]

Shortly after the Anderson report, on June 1, 1960, officials from Methodist Hospital gathered to break ground for a $9 million, 375-bed expansion. This new wing would provide larger surgical facilities and raise Methodist Hospital's total bed capacity to approximately 700. On June 3, 1960, Sue Vaughan Clayton, Will Clayton's wife, donated 124,000 shares of stock in Anderson, Clayton & Company, worth a reported $4.5 million, to create an endowment for Texas Children's Hospital, the largest single grant received by the medical center up to that time. On June 30, St. Luke's Episcopal Hospital announced that it was launching a drive to raise $9 million for a building expansion program. And in September the board of regents of the University of Texas approved a $4.3 million addition to the M. D. Anderson Hospital and Tumor Institute to provide more space for research. Amid all of this activity, the executive director of the Texas Medical Center, Frederick Elliott, could only conclude, "This year, 1960, has been a most satisfactory one." The year had been important for Houston in the area of civil rights, too. Although people often think of Houston's Western heritage, it was equally influenced by Southern mores, including Jim Crow laws mandating racial segregation. Compared with other Southern cities, however, the civil rights movement in Houston generally was a less violent, more civil campaign. On December 26, 1956, the NAACP helped file a lawsuit to desegregate the Houston Independent School District. On March 4, 1960, students from the historically black Texas Southern University organized the city's first sit-in protest. Not wishing to let the protests spiral into violence, on September 1, 1960, nine major downtown businesses quietly desegregated their lunch counters. And on September 8, the first African American student enrolled at a previously all-white public school. In the Texas Medical Center institutions complied with the deeply entrenched laws and traditions of the racially segregated South and dealt with desegregation on an individual basis. The University of Texas Dental Branch actually had been among the first to admit African American students in 1952, when Zeb Poindexter and Moritz Virano Craven matriculated. As new institutions opened in the medical center, they frequently made provisions for treating patients without regard to race or creed. But although the old laws and customs would fall in time, racially segregated facilities and staff continued for many years.[28]

By contrast, 1961 was relatively calm. But as the end of the year approached, officials from the city of Houston and Harris County announced that, at long last, they had reached an agreement to build the new city-county hospital in the Texas Medical Center. Elliott had supported the creation of the hospital for many years, but in his role as executive director of the medical center, he wisely opted to refrain from the sometimes rancorous debate that had split Houston's medical community. Many doctors and concerned citizens worried about building the new charity hospital in the Texas Medical Center; they were concerned that it would be too far from the neighborhoods where most of Houston's poor resided and would thus be ineffective. Others worried that by having doctors and medical students from Baylor University College of Medicine staff the hospital, somehow tax dollars would be supporting a private medical college. In the end, city-county politics and disputes among the doctors of the Harris County Medical Society dragged out the argument for more than a decade. But when groundbreaking ceremonies finally took place, officials announced that the hospital would be named Ben Taub General Hospital, in honor of Ben Taub, a Houston businessman and philanthropist who had served as chairman of Jefferson Davis Hospital from 1935 to 1964. Taub, a life-long bachelor with a tremendous gift of compassion, gave many volunteer hours to visiting patients at "Jeff Davis." He also had a major role in the DePelchin Faith Home for homeless children as well as the United Way charity and served on the board of trustees of the Texas Medical Center. Taub donated thirty-five acres of land to the University of Houston, provided funds for scholarships, and subsidized visiting medical professors. Ben Taub General Hospital would open in May of 1963 and in time became known as one of the nation's leading trauma centers.[29]

Early in 1962 Fred Elliott met with Leland Anderson and announced his plans to retire. As he wrote in his memoir, "I told him that it was my

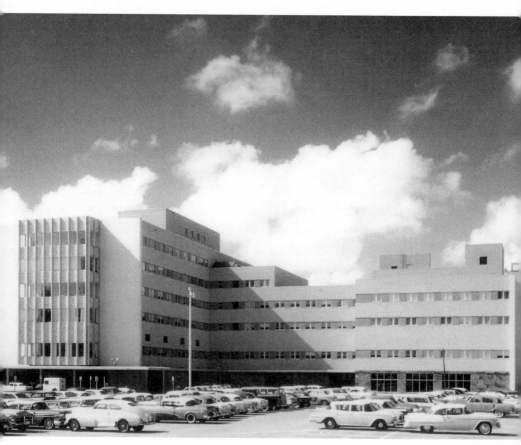

*Ben Taub Hospital, ca. 1963. Courtesy of John P. McGovern Historical Collections and Research Center, Texas Medical Center Library.*

feeling that the Medical Center was entering into a period that would require the energies of one much younger than I." Elliott suggested a change of title for the new head of the medical center to executive vice president, which would better describe the position and fit more appropriately with the administrative structures of the other institutions. The search for the new executive vice president began immediately. During the spring, the board appointed Dr. Richard T. Eastwood to succeed Dr. Elliott. At the time, Eastwood was vice president of business operations at the University of Alabama in Birmingham, where the school's medical center was located. His administrative and educational background made him a perfect candidate for the position at the Texas Medical Center. He was to begin his appointment on August 15, 1962.[30]

In May the board of trustees elected new officers for the medical center. They reelected Leland Anderson as president and William B. Bates, Hines Baker, and Frederick C. Elliott as vice presidents; Dr. Eastwood, who attended the meeting, was formally appointed executive vice president and elected secretary of the board of trustees. William Kirkland and Carroll Simmons were reelected as treasurer and assistant treasurer, respectively. On July 31, 1962, Elliott presented his final agenda to the medical center's board of trustees. He had agreed to stay on to assist Eastwood in a development role. But by the following spring, it became clear that having the former director present in the office was an awkward arrangement, and Elliott resigned as an employee effective May 31, 1963. With Ben Taub General Hospital having opened earlier in the month, it was a fitting time for him to step aside.

Elliott's retirement as director marked the end of an important period in the development of the Texas Medical Center. Many Houstonians and people around the country recognized his role during this formative period, and John H. Freeman credited E. W. Bertner for bringing Elliott into the Texas Medical Center. "Bertner knew Fred Elliott," said Freeman years later. "And when he found it was possible to get the Texas Dental College into the University [of Texas] System and to take Fred Elliott as part of the package, plans were abandoned to bring Baylor Dental College from Dallas. Elliott had a reputation as a fine man and educator. And the fact that he was a part of the Texas Dental [College] made it a most attractive opportunity to the trustees and to Bertner."[31]

When Richard Eastwood took over as executive vice president of the Texas Medical Center, it signaled the end of the foundational years for the medical center and the beginning of a new period of development. Not only was it a well-established and highly esteemed facility, its institutions continued to expand as the numbers of patients treated grew and new staff were hired. During the next fifty years of its history, the Texas Medical Center would grow to a point where it was renowned worldwide as one of the leading centers for medical education, research, and patient care. In all of this, one of the major forces driving the development of the Texas Medical Center and its growing number of institutions was the M. D. Anderson Foundation. In fact, it can safely be said that the Anderson Foundation played an indispensable part in creating and nurturing the Texas Medical Center, and in the process it succeeded in fulfilling Monroe D. Anderson's wishes far beyond what even his creative mind might have envisioned.

# Chapter 9

## *The Biggest Medical Center in the World*

Fifty years after the end of what has been characterized as its "founding era" in 1962, the Texas Medical Center is today recognized as the largest medical complex in the world. The number of institutions that formally joined the Texas Medical Center had increased from a handful during the formative years to over fifty by 2012. As the Texas Medical Center continued to add new member institutions, the board of trustees approved construction of a host of new buildings, acquired more land, and developed plans to accommodate the continuing growth. Although it is beyond the scope of this book to present a detailed history of all the institutions that make up the Texas Medical Center, a general overview here will illustrate both the extraordinary success of this medical complex and the lasting legacy of Monroe D. Anderson through the work of his philanthropic foundation as a driving force behind the medical center.

### Texas Medical Center, Inc.

Although the founders envisioned a medical center in which all of the institutions would function together in a collaborative, cooperative manner, the increasing number and diversity of institutions has made this an unrealistic goal for many years. But throughout its history the corporate body, Texas Medical Center, Inc. (TMC), known today simply as Texas Medical Center, has maintained continuing interaction with all of its member institutions. TMC, ostensibly, is like "city hall" in what is a "city of health" with a number of responsibilities including enforcing the covenants and maintaining streets, common areas, parking, and other aspects of infrastructure. Generally though, the individual member institutions have functioned independently of each other. During these years, TMC continued to purchase additional land as nearby tracts became available, and in 1981 lands that the University of Texas had acquired on its own also became part of the center. In 1985 the medical center added the old Shamrock Hilton Hotel and its 22.6 acres of land to its inventory. But the iconic old building proved too expensive to rehabilitate and was torn down a few years later to make way for parking. This pattern of land acquisition continued; by 2012 the Texas Medical Center had grown to some 1,300 acres of land with 280 buildings providing 45.5 million square feet of space.[1]

In addition to attracting many of the best and brightest physicians and students to its main campus, the Texas Medical Center also benefited from having talented leadership for its corporate structure. TMC enjoyed a long period of stable leadership under Richard Eastwood's tenure from 1962 to 1980. When Eastwood died in 1980, Jack Kenney Williams, the former president and chancellor of Texas A&M University, was appointed as his successor. But Williams died suddenly just a few months after taking the helm. The board of trustees then turned to former University of Houston president Philip G. Hoffman, who served as president until November 1984, when the trustees chose Richard E. Wainerdi, who took over as president and chief executive officer. Leadership of the board of trustees followed a similar path, with Leland Anderson continuing as chairman until he retired in 1976. The board then chose attorney Herman P. Pressler, who served for the next five years. He was followed by attorney Leon Jaworski (1981–82), newspaper publisher Richard J. V. Johnson (1983–86), and attorney William C. Harvin (1986–92). In 1992 the board then chose Houston businessman David M. Underwood as chairman, and his tenure has continued to the present, providing steady, stable leadership. For over twenty years, then, with Richard Wainerdi as president and CEO and David Underwood as chairman of the board, the Texas Medical Center experienced a period of consistency in its direction—from men whose ideas about the concept of the medical center reflected the goals of the original founders—to build a "city of health" in Houston. Their leadership skills enabled them to guide the Texas Medical Center through a series of catastrophic weather events and institutional challenges to become the largest medical complex in the world.

It was during the late 1960s, however, that the original spirit of cooperation among the institutions of the medical center seemed to be rejuvenated, however slightly, when discussions led to the establishment of two important entities through which the medical center's institutions could cooperate: Thermal Energy Corporation and the Hospital Laundry Cooperative Association. In 1968 Houston Natural Gas

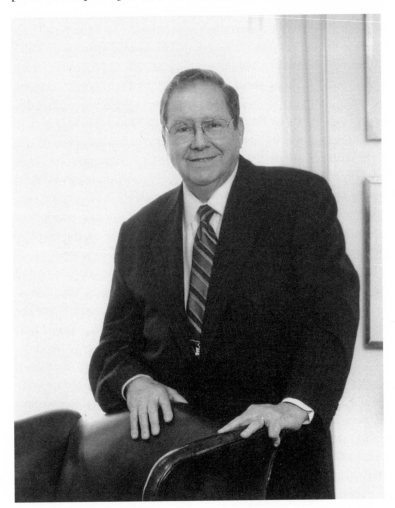

*Richard E. Wainerdi, president of the Texas Medical Center from 1984 to 2013. Photo by Kaye Marvins Photography, Inc.; courtesy of Texas Medical Center.*

Corporation built the Texas Medical Center's central heating and cooling plant on the land between Holcombe Boulevard and Brays Bayou. The plant was designed to provide chilled water for air-conditioning and steam for heat and other uses. This central plant eliminated both the need for each building it served to have its own cooling system and boilers and also the requisite hiring of professional staff to run these climate control systems. Nine years later, several institutions of the Texas Medical Center formed a nonprofit, cooperative association and purchased the plant, and in 1978 the Texas Medical Center Central Heating and Cooling Services Cooperative Association, now known as Thermal Energy Corporation (TECO), became a member institution of TMC. Over the years, TECO expanded its capacity as demand increased from the growth of the Texas Medical Center. By 2011 TECO was the largest district energy company in the United States and one of the leading district energy firms in the world. Around the same time as TECO began, in 1970 planning began to build a central laundry facility as a cooperative that all institutions of the Texas Medical Center could join. The Texas Medical Center Hospital Laundry Cooperative Association was built on land next to TECO. In 2006 the laundry relocated to a larger, state-of-the-art facility, and the old building was demolished to make way for the TECO expansion. In these two co-ops, then, the vision of the medical center's founders for a collaborative community found new life.[2]

Despite the cooperative goodwill generated by creating TECO and the laundry, other challenges arose to confront this collegial spirit. Most notably, during May 1996, the Texas Medical Center faced a situation that threatened the very core concept upon which it was built: that only not-for-profit institutions could become members and build on TMC land. During the 1990s hospitals around the country were consolidating and seeking alliances in order to survive in the competitive new world of managed care. Columbia HCA Healthcare Corporation and St. Luke's Episcopal Hospital had been in serious discussions about an affiliation, an agreement that would have given the for-profit Columbia HCA a foothold in the medical center. In order to protect the medical center's nonprofit status, TMC filed suit against St. Luke's, stating that the proposed alliance between the two hospitals would constitute a violation of the deed restrictions that prohibited any for-profit activity in the medical center. In fact, St. Luke's had agreed to abide by these restrictions in 1951 when it first accepted land to build its hospital in the Texas Medical Center.[3]

Hospital officials and other leaders in Houston's health care community believed that if the deal between St. Luke's and Columbia/HCA was finalized, it would set a precedent and other similar agreements would quickly follow, destroying the medical center as a nonprofit, health-centered complex. The threat posed by an affiliation between St. Luke's and Columbia HCA became more apparent when news surfaced of meetings between David Page, the president and chief executive officer of Hermann Hospital, and officials from the Nashville-based OrNda Healthcorp. OrNda had already signed an agreement with the Memorial Healthcare System regarding the Houston Northwest Medical Center and began to focus on securing an alliance with a hospital in the Texas Medical Center, a move that would improve its competitive position as a managed care network. If the St. Luke's and Columbia HCA deal went through, it might open the way for Hermann/OrNda and other institutions in the medical center to follow suit.[4]

But in the end, the TMC covenants, originally drafted by John H. Freeman, withstood the challenge.[5] In late August 1996, Judge Carolyn Clause Garcia of the 151st Judicial District Court found the deed restrictions to be "valid and enforceable," which prompted St. Luke's and TMC to reach an out-of-court settlement.[6] In the aftermath of the lawsuit, the TMC board of directors agreed to form a committee to oversee similar proposals from any of the member institutions in the future. With the potential for mergers with for-profit companies quashed by the courts and the Texas attorney general, on July 1, 1997, two revered local nonprofit hospital systems, Hermann Hospital and Memorial Healthcare System, announced that they would join together. On November 4, 1997, they formally created the Memorial Hermann Healthcare System.[7]

Meanwhile, with the St. Luke's and Columbia HCA lawsuit behind them, TMC officials initiated a new master planning program, working with consultants and with other organizations, including TECO, METRO, and the Friends of Hermann Park. In 1999 TMC unveiled its "Fifty-year Master Plan" for the central campus and recommended that the member institutions incorporate these guidelines into their own plans for future development. During the year, TMC also began exploring ideas to create a research park on land south of the main campus that would include the University of Texas M. D. Anderson Cancer Center, the University of Texas Health Science Center at Houston, and Baylor College of Medicine. TMC also developed plans for what was described as a "Central Campus Amenities Building, Garage and Plaza," near the center of the main campus. Years earlier, Frederick Elliott had imagined a "commons" building that would serve as a gathering place for medical students, staff, patients, and visitors to the Texas Medical Center. That dream was fulfilled on October 4, 2002, with the opening of the Texas Medical Center John P. McGovern Commons. The eye-catching new structure featured an above-grade parking garage disguised behind two sixty-foot water walls, a ground-level food court and plaza, and, above the garage, a restaurant and conference space with a sweeping view of the medical center. In 2000, while construction was under way on the commons building, TMC purchased the twenty-two-acre Nabisco bakery facility at Holcombe Boulevard and Almeda. TMC renovated the historic 600,000-square-foot building as research, office, and classroom space, renting some of it to member institutions and developing new administrative offices in the building. On December 9, 2005, TMC formally moved its corporate offices from the Jesse H. Jones Library Building to the Nabisco facility, renamed the Texas Medical Center John P. McGovern Campus. The commons and the new campus were named to honor Dr. John P. McGovern, a Houston allergist and philanthropist who was a longtime supporter of many worthy causes related to the Texas Medical Center. This adaptive reuse and renovation of the historic old building won several awards, including the 2005 Good Brick Award presented by Preservation Houston.[8]

While all of this expansion and construction was under way, local officials began taking steps to protect the expanding medical center from the frequent flooding that occurred when nearby Brays Bayou overflowed its banks. In 2000 the Harris County Commissioners Court approved the $229 million Brays Bayou Flood Control Project. The plan was scheduled to take eight to ten years to complete and would help relieve the damaging impact of flooding in the Texas Medical Center. Because hurricanes and tropical storms are fairly common in the area and drainage is problematic due to the flat terrain, flooding remained a continuing challenge both in the Texas Medical Center and throughout the city of Houston.[9]

But the work on the Brays Bayou project was just getting under way when on June 8, 2001, wind currents pushing Tropical Storm Allison, which had passed through Houston three days earlier, caused the storm to circle back to pour an additional three feet of rain on the already-saturated city. The massive flooding from the storm caused damage to more than 70,000 homes, killed twenty-two people, and inflicted approximately $5 billion in damages, including substantial ruin in the Texas Medical Center. Many buildings lost power, basements flooded, and Hermann Hospital had to call for volunteers and helicopters to help evacuate patients from the darkened building. At the University of Texas Medical School–Houston, an estimated ten million gallons of water poured into the basement and flooded the ground floor. The flood destroyed research animals and ruined medical equipment, files, and crucial records. It took a full month, and much longer in some cases, for the affected institutions to complete the necessary cleanup and repairs in order to reopen. The storm prompted officials to take more drastic measures to prevent or minimize similar damage from future storms. It also demonstrated the resilience of the city and the institutions of the Texas Medical Center. Just four years later, in the aftermath of Hurricane Katrina and the devastation it inflicted on New Orleans, Houston mayor Bill White and Harris County judge Robert Eckels opened the Houston Astrodome and the George R. Brown Convention Center as shelters for refugees from the storm. The Harris County Hospital District, in concert with a host of city, county, and Texas Medical Center officials, Baylor College of Medicine, the Michael E. DeBakey Veterans Affairs Medical Center (MEDVACM), and the University of Texas Health Science Center at Houston established two medical communities at these shelters. This monumental effort provided medical services and other assistance to nearly 25,000 Hurricane Katrina evacuees.[10]

In 2008 emergency planning and flood prevention measures put in place after Tropical Storm Allison were put to the test when Hurricane Ike, a strong Category 2 hurricane, made landfall at Galveston early in the morning of Saturday, September 13. Hurricane-force winds extended 120 miles from the center of the storm, which damaged office buildings and homes, knocked down trees and power lines, and cut electric power to nearly the entire Houston metropolitan area and an estimated 4.5 million customers in Southeast Texas. The storm surge and rain flooded some 100,000 homes and left Galveston uninhabitable for weeks. Hurricane Ike took at least 112 lives in its path across the United States, including thirty-seven known victims in Texas. Although electric power was out in most of the region, the lights remained on at the Texas Medical Center, and power was restored in much of the downtown by Saturday evening. Most of the electrical distribution lines on the medical center's main campus had been buried underground and protected from winds, falling trees, and other hurricane hazards. However, the Mid-Campus, home to MEDVACM, and the John P. McGovern Campus, located across the street at Holcombe and Almeda, both lost power, since the lines there were aboveground. But the county's flood prevention efforts proved successful, and the turbulent waters raging down Brays Bayou remained within its banks. There was some minor street flooding in the medical center, but it quickly drained away. "The lesson learned here," said TMC president Richard Wainerdi, "is that those drainage projects, though they at times caused headaches for motorists, worked well to protect the Texas Medical Center from possible flooding."[11]

In addition to its drainage improvements, land acquisitions, and infrastructure maintenance, one of the most significant initiatives of the Texas Medical Center in recent years has been centered on encouraging research—the creation of the National Center for Human Performance (NCHP). The idea behind forming the center was to support participation by scholars and practitioners in the United States and from around the world in studying human performance in four primary areas: physical and artistic development, individual and team sports, space exploration, and military endeavors. Planning began in 2003, and within two years TMC gained the support of sixteen member institutions that signed a memorandum of understanding supporting its efforts to establish the NCHP. By 2006 twenty-two institutions had signed affiliation agreements, and the following year the NCHP opened in the John P. McGovern Campus. In 2010 the US Congress enacted legislation that included appropriations of about $665.8 million "to advance science and research on human performance in space, health, the military, athletics, and the arts." The bill also assigned the prestigious Designation as Institution of Excellence to the NCHP, an institution that Congress recognized as being "dedicated to understanding and improving all aspects of human performance."[12]

Over the years, then, the Texas Medical Center has worked to provide a setting in which its existing institutions could thrive and in which new institutions could become successful members of an entity totally dedicated to human health. And during this period the M. D. Anderson Foundation continued its support of the medical center and the institutions that it comprises. It is important to look briefly at some of the milestones in the development and expansion of these institutions over time to appreciate fully how the Texas Medical Center grew to become the largest medical complex in the world.

## M. D. Anderson Hospital and Tumor Institute

The University of Texas M. D. Anderson Hospital and Tumor Institute was the first of the original institutions in what became the Texas Medical Center. From its humble beginnings on the grounds of the old Baker estate, the cancer hospital carried out its mission in a spectacular way becoming one of the most highly regarded in the world and consistently rated as the top cancer center in the United States. One of the first steps in achieving this recognition occurred following the passage of the National Cancer Act of 1971. As a result of this legislation, the M. D. Anderson Hospital and Tumor Institute was designated as one of the first three Comprehensive Cancer Centers in the country. This designation also attracted more patients, which in turn increased the need for more space. The hospital continued to build and in 1976 opened a chapel, a radio-therapy center, a new clinic building, and the Lutheran Hospital Pavilion, doubling the size of the hospital's physical plant. During the next decade, more buildings followed, including the R. E. "Bob" Smith Research Building and the R. Lee Clark Clinic. The hospital had evolved into more of a cancer research and treatment complex over the years, and in 1988 the University of Texas board of regents approved a name change to the University of Texas M. D. Anderson Cancer Center, which better reflected the nature of the institution. In 1993 the M. D. Anderson Cancer Center began another era of construction that continued almost nonstop for the next twenty years. Along with the construction of new research, hospital, and ambulatory care facilities, the cancer center opened the Jesse H. Jones Rotary House International, a specialty hotel for patients and families from out of town to stay during treatment visits. The hotel was connected to the cancer center by a sky bridge over busy Holcombe Boulevard. More buildings were constructed, and with open space becoming scarce on the main campus by 2007, the University of Texas acquired some 110 acres—the University of Texas Research Park—that would become known as the Texas Medical Center South Campus. Here the cancer center began construction of the Center for Advanced Biomedical Imaging Research, a joint project with the University of Texas Health Science Center at Houston and General Electric Healthcare.

## Baylor College of Medicine

Baylor University College of Medicine holds the distinction of being the first institution to construct and open a building on the medical center campus (1948). As discussed in the previous chapter, in 1959 the medical college formed a unique partnership with TMC, which acquired federal funds on behalf of the school to construct three badly needed new buildings. In 1964 Baylor University College of Medicine and the Texas Medical Center dedicated these three new buildings that were the result of their unique collaboration—the M. D. Anderson Basic Science Building, the Jewish Institute for Medical Research, and the Jesse H. Jones Clinical Research Building. Four years later, on November 13, 1968, Baylor University College of Medicine reached an agreement to separate from Baylor University in order to make it possible for the renamed Baylor College of Medicine to apply for and receive financial assistance from the government.[13] During the next four decades Baylor College of Medicine added several new buildings to its campus within the heart of the Texas Medical Center, including the Michael E. DeBakey Center for Biomedical Education and Research, the R. E. "Bob" and Vivian Smith Medical Research Building, and, in the late 1990s, the sixteen-story Albert B. Alkek School of Biomedical Sciences at Baylor College of Medicine. And in what could be described as a coup for the Texas Medical Center, in 2001 Baylor College of Medicine and Methodist Hospital formed a partnership to bring the famed Menninger Clinic, known as one of the nation's leading psychiatric hospitals, from Topeka, Kansas, to Houston. The clinic moved into an existing facility in northwest Houston in 2003; on April 12, 2012, it opened a new 120-bed, 161,000-square-foot hospital on a fifty-acre tract on South Main

Street, closer to the Texas Medical Center. This "mental health epicenter" was designed to support future advancements in mental health treatment, prevention, and research and also to encourage collaboration among researchers and scientists in the Texas Medical Center and on a national and international basis.[14]

## A Second Medical School

During the late 1960s, as the M. D. Anderson Cancer Center continued to grow, the University of Texas increased its presence in the Texas Medical Center with the founding of the University of Texas Medical School at Houston. To meet the growing demand for more physicians in the state, in 1969 the Texas Legislature established the University of Texas Medical School at Houston. This set off yet another flurry of activity in the Texas Medical Center, as the university signed an affiliation agreement with Hermann Hospital to be its primary teaching hospital, began a search for a dean, and started the planning process to construct the needed buildings. In January 1970 the university appointed Dr. Cheves M. Smyth as founding dean and later in the year enrolled the first class of nineteen students. Since no buildings yet existed for the new medical school, these students began taking classes at other University of Texas locations. The Texas Medical Center allocated 5.5 acres of land for the new medical school, which would be located adjacent to the library and to Hermann Hospital. In 1972 the medical school completed its first building on the campus, named in honor of John H. Freeman. Planning continued for construction of a larger medical school building that would be contiguous with the new Jesse H. Jones Pavilion of Hermann Hospital. In addition, the board of regents approved the creation of an umbrella organizational structure, the University of Texas Health Science Center at Houston. Known today simply as UTHealth, it includes the schools of dentistry, nursing, public health, and biomedical informatics; the medical school; and the Graduate School of Biomedical Sciences. Harkening back to the days of Dr. Lee Clark, the University of Texas M. D. Anderson Cancer Center remains independent of UTHealth. After delays caused by flood damage in 1976, the main building of the University of Texas Medical School was completed and opened in 1977.[15]

Four years later, in 1981, the Texas Legislature created the Harris County Psychiatric Center. The psychiatric center broke ground for its new facility on South MacGregor in 1984 and admitted its first patient in October 1986. In 1990 it formally became a unit of UTHealth and today is known as the University of Texas Harris County Psychiatric Center. Over time, the schools of UTHealth continued to attract talented faculty and grow in reputation. This in turn attracted more students and researchers. As the twentieth century faded into history, a new wave of expansion swept the Texas Medical Center, including its medical schools. In 2001, after Tropical Storm Allison dropped over three feet of rain on Houston, many UTHealth buildings and laboratories

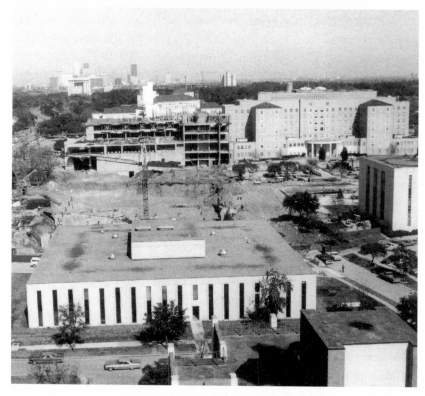

*University of Texas Medical School at Houston under construction, 1975. Pictured are the John H. Freeman Building (foreground); the site of the main building, marked by a construction crane; and the unfinished Jesse H. Jones Pavilion of Hermann Hospital (background). Downtown Houston is seen in the distance. Courtesy of John P. McGovern Historical Collections and Research Center, Texas Medical Center Library.*

were devastated. Repairs began immediately, but the Freeman Building was deemed too badly damaged and was demolished. New construction began, including an $80 million, six-story research facility on the site of the old Freeman Building. In 2006, with the new medical school building under construction, the board of regents of the University of Texas System allocated $77.1 million to fund two new construction projects in the Texas Medical Center, a biomedical research and education center as a home for adult stem cell research and teaching and a new building for the University of Texas Dental Branch at Houston. In 2008 the lobby in the new building of the University of Texas Medical School at Houston was named in honor of John H. Freeman. Since it was first created, the medical school has trained over 5,000 physicians in addition to residency, fellow training, and continuing education programs.[16]

## Other Educational and Research Institutions

In addition to Baylor College of Medicine and the University of Texas Health Science Center at Houston, other health-related educational institutions sought to join as member institutions in the growing complex of the Texas Medical Center. Some of these schools included Texas Women's University (TWU), Houston Community College (HCC), Prairie View A&M University College of Nursing, the University of Houston (UH), Texas Southern University (TSU), and Texas A&M University. Texas Women's University first began offering classes in Houston in 1961 and opened its Mary Gibbs Jones Hall in 1969. This allowed TWU to double its facilities for training in nursing, occupational therapy, and physical therapy and to add new interdisciplinary laboratories. Nearly forty years later, in 2006, the school replaced its aging facility and opened the TWU Institute of Health Sciences–Houston Center, a modern ten-story, 202,000-square-foot, environmentally friendly "campus in one building."[17] Also during the 1970s HCC began offering degreed programs in health science. The programs flourished over the years with the result that in 1999 HCC centralized the location of its various health programs at the John B. Coleman Health Science Center on the HCC Southeast College campus. By 2004, the program had expanded to offer twenty-one degrees and certificates in health science fields. In

1978 Prairie View A&M College of Nursing established an RN-Bachelor of Science in Nursing program in Houston. Four years later, the college moved into facilities on Fannin Street and formally became a member institution. Since then, Prairie View A&M University College of Nursing has established a Master of Science Family Nurse Practitioner program and, in January 2005, an LVN-BSN program. In 2006 the nursing school moved into a new state-of-the-art facility on Fannin Street with enough space to accommodate an anticipated future enrollment of between 500 to 600 upper-division and graduate students.[18] In 1980 the UH College of Pharmacy became a member institution and moved into its own building on the Texas Medical Center campus. In 2004 UH and Methodist Hospital formed an academic partnership as UH expanded its research programs in health-related fields. In 2009 UH as a whole became an official member institution and created a new biomedical engineering department in its Cullen College of Engineering. The university began construction of a new, six-story, 167,000-square-foot Health and Biomedical Sciences Center (HBSC) on its main campus to house the new department. While UH was taking its early steps into health research, in 1984 TSU launched a Doctor of Pharmacy program, and in 2001 the TSU College of Pharmacy and Health Sciences became a member institution of Texas Medical Center. In 1986 Texas A&M University established its Institute of Biosciences and Technology in the Texas Medical Center (now known as Texas A&M University Health Science Center Institute of Biosciences and Technology) and became a member institution. Three years later Texas A&M began construction of an eleven-story Institute of Biosciences and Technology Research and Education facility, which opened in 1992. Finally, although Rice University had been involved with the Texas Medical Center from the beginning, in 2003 it formally became a member institution.[19]

In another educational endeavor that was unique to the Texas Medical Center, in 1972 the Houston Independent School District (HISD) and Baylor College of Medicine teamed up to open the first High School for Health Professions (HSHP) in the nation. The school, which held classes on the Baylor campus, became a member institution in 1973. HSHP offered a demanding, comprehensive, precollege program for students with interests in health care, medicine, and the sciences that included opportunities to gain hands-on experience in the facilities of the Texas Medical Center. Enrollment quickly grew to 200 students in 1973 and to 450 in 1975. Realizing that it had a burgeoning success, in 1978 HISD acquired a four-acre tract of land near the medical center and began construction on a new building for the high school. In 1996 the school was renamed the Michael E. DeBakey High School for Health Professions, and it continues to be rated among the best overall high schools and a perennial leader in math and science in the country.[20]

## A Third Medical School

One of the most significant events in the history of the Texas Medical Center occurred on March 2, 2010, with the announcement that the University of Texas Medical Branch at Galveston (UTMB) would become the forty-ninth member institution of the Texas Medical Center. TMC's president and CEO, Richard E. Wainerdi, spoke about the potential for greater collaboration that the medical center's newest member would bring when he said at a news conference, "As a member of the Texas Medical Center, UTMB will be collaborating more closely with other member institutions, and this relationship will further increase the combined level of expertise that will be a material benefit to citizens throughout Texas and beyond." During this news conference, UTMB president Dr. David L. Callender expressed a similar sentiment about the historic affiliation: "We are honored to become the newest member of such a highly-regarded organization. Collaboration is a key to expanding excellence among Texas Medical Center institutions and, ultimately, our collective ability to address the health needs of a rapidly growing region. While Galveston will always be UTMB's home, the people we serve will benefit as we strengthen connections with fellow Texas Medical Center institutions to ensure the Houston/Galveston region remains a leader in health sciences education, research and patient care well into the future." Thus, nearly eighty years after Will and Mike Hogg first purchased the original 134-acre tract of land, hoping to lure UTMB to move to Houston, the state's oldest medical school had finally joined the Texas Medical Center. But it did so on its own terms and maintained its home base in Galveston, where it had been training the state's physicians and health care professionals since 1891.[21]

## Hospitals in the Texas Medical Center

One of the most significant changes in Houston-area health care occurred in November 1965, when voters in Harris County approved creation of the Harris County Hospital District (HCHD) to make medical care available for all residents of the county. Two months later, on January 1, 1966, the newly formed HCHD formally took ownership of the two existing city-county hospitals, Jefferson Davis and Ben Taub. By 2012, the district had grown to fourteen community health centers, eight school-based clinics, a dental and dialysis center, several mobile health units, and the Quentin R. Mease Community Hospital, which had become a member institution of the Texas Medical Center in 1986. Also in 1986 the HCHD broke ground for a new 578-bed Ben Taub General Hospital next door to the original building and also began construction on the new Lyndon B. Johnson General Hospital (LBJ), intended to replace the aging facilities at Jefferson Davis Hospital. Three years later, in 1989, HCHD opened the new 328-bed LBJ General Hospital in northeast Houston, which immediately became a member institution of the Texas Medical Center, and closed the old Jeff Davis Hospital on Allen Parkway. Shortly after LBJ Hospital opened, the University of Texas Medical School at Houston reached an affiliation agreement with HCHD to provide medical staff to LBJ Hospital and five of the district's community health centers. Today HCHD, now known as Harris Health System (as of September 6, 2012), is a teaching facility for Baylor College of Medicine and for the schools of UTHealth.[22]

Hermann Hospital remained a private institution and languished for much of the 1960s until the 1969 affiliation agreement to become the primary teaching hospital for the new University of Texas Medical School at Houston. The coming of the new medical school prompted construction and renovations for Hermann Hospital. The new Jesse H. and Mary Gibbs Jones Pavilion, constructed so as to be contiguous with the medical school building, opened in 1977. While it was under construction, in 1973, the John S. Dunn Helistop at Hermann Hospital opened to provide emergency air ambulance service and medical care for patients in the surrounding area. The new helistop helped inspire Dr. James "Red" Duke, medical director of Hermann Hospital's Emergency Center and a professor of surgery at the new University of Texas

Medical School, to launch the first air ambulance service in Texas—Life Flight—at Hermann Hospital. By 1996 Life Flight had flown over 50,000 missions. Today Memorial Hermann Life Flight provides critical care and air medical transport service for emergency patients within a 150-mile radius of the Texas Medical Center. Life Flight has grown from one leased helicopter to six state-of-the-art helicopters and a crew that includes thirteen pilots, fourteen flight nurses, fifteen paramedics/dispatchers, and five mechanics. Since its inaugural flight in 1976, Memorial Hermann Life Flight has flown more than 120,000 missions to date. Because of the growing expertise of its trauma center doctors and the sterling reputation of its Life Flight program, in 1994 Hermann Hospital was designated as the first Level 1 Trauma Center in Houston. In 1997 Hermann Hospital merged with the Memorial Healthcare System, creating the Memorial Hermann Healthcare System. During the years since the merger, the hospital (now known as Memorial Hermann-TMC) has thrived and in 2007 opened the thirty-story Memorial Hermann Medical Plaza in partnership with Mischer Healthcare. This was followed in March 2008 by the new, 230,000-square-foot Memorial Hermann Heart and Vascular Institute.[23]

On May 29, 2012, Memorial Hermann-TMC made history again with the announcement that it would establish the Texas Trauma Institute, designed to improve survival and recovery rates for trauma victims. The new institute, affiliated with UTHealth's medical school, would bring together the best researchers, physicians, and educators to develop new treatments and protocols designed to improve quality of life for trauma patients. The Texas Trauma Institute brought in as director one of the military's finest surgeons, Col. John B. Holcomb. The institute provides some 200 beds and twenty-four-hour emergency and trauma care to patients, who also have access to TIRR Memorial Hermann. TIRR, formerly the Texas Institute for Rehabilitation and Research, had become highly renowned since it first opened in the medical center in 1959. TIRR constructed new additions in 1965 and again in 1974 and in 1991 opened the Edna B. Dunn Tower. Over the years, having "Texas" in its name caused the institute to be confused as being a state agency, so in 1978 TIRR changed its name to The Institute for Rehabilitation and Research. In 2006 TIRR reached an agreement with Memorial Hermann Healthcare System to consolidate services and form TIRR Memorial Hermann, further enhancing the reputations of both institutions.[24]

While Hermann Hospital was growing in size and renown, so too was Methodist Hospital, St. Luke's Episcopal Hospital, and Texas Children's Hospital. In 1963 Methodist Hospital opened a new, 180-bed annex and continued to construct new facilities over the years, including the Fondren and Brown Orthopedic and Cardiovascular Centers, Alkek Tower, Scurlock Tower, and the twenty-six-story Smith Tower. In 2004 the hospital created the Methodist Neurological Institute and, after a dispute with Baylor College of Medicine, began a new affiliation with Weill Cornell Medical College for training residents and conducting research. During this same period of time, St. Luke's Episcopal Hospital and Texas Children's Hospital opened a twenty-seven-story expansion in 1969 that increased the total bed capacity to over 1,300 beds, followed by a twenty-six-story patient tower in 1971. The joint governance between the two hospitals ended in 1987 when they signed a formal separation agreement, making each hospital independent. St. Luke's continued to grow and in 1990 opened the distinctive St. Luke's Medical Tower (known today as the O'Quinn Medical Tower at St. Luke's). As their reputations for providing quality health care grew, both of these pioneer hospitals of the Texas Medical Center continued to attract more patients and many of the nation's finest physicians.[25]

In addition to their hospital services, both Methodist and St. Luke's developed highly renowned cardiac care centers led by two of the greatest heart surgeons of the twentieth century, Drs. Michael E. DeBakey and Denton A. Cooley. Denton Cooley had grown up in Houston and trained at UTMB and at Johns Hopkins. He had returned to Houston in 1951 to work out of Baylor University College of Medicine and Methodist Hospital as a heart surgeon with Michael DeBakey. In 1962, after several years and a series of disagreements with DeBakey, Cooley set out to establish a cardiac surgery program of his own and chartered the Texas Heart Institute. During the next fifty years, the rivalry between the two cardiac surgeons generated a competition that helped fuel research into heart transplant surgery and the development of artificial heart technology. Both Methodist and St. Luke's became known worldwide through their affiliations with these two great cardiac surgeons and in the process enhanced the reputation of the Texas Medical Center as a place for research and training as well as patient care. In 2001 the Texas Heart Institute at St. Luke's performed its 100,000th open-heart operation. In that same year the Methodist DeBakey Heart and Vascular Center officially opened. The following year the Denton A. Cooley Building of the Texas Heart Institute opened. The two surgeons reconciled in October 2007, just nine months before DeBakey died, at age ninety-nine, on July 11, 2008.[26]

Texas Children's Hospital also continued to thrive and in 1967 doubled the number of rooms to some 222. In 1991 Texas Children's Hospital became the nation's largest freestanding pediatric hospital when it completed an expansion that brought its licensed bed total to 456. Another expansion in 2003 brought the total number of licensed beds to 715 and saw the addition of a Ronald McDonald House on the fourth floor of the hospital's original building, renamed the Abercrombie Building in honor of longtime patron James S. Abercrombie. This Ronald McDonald House provides twenty overnight sleeping rooms for families with children in the pediatric intensive care unit and the neonatal Level 2 nursery. In 2008 Texas Children's Hospital and Baylor College of Medicine teamed up to extend their reach to Africa with the opening of a 21,000-square-foot clinical care center, the Baylor International Pediatric AIDS Initiative at Texas Children's Hospital (BIPAI) in Kampala, Uganda. On its opening day, BIPAI received some 6,000 transfer patients and instantly became the world's largest pediatric HIV/AIDS center. Texas Children's Hospital continued to expand its presence in Houston with the 2010 opening of the Jan and Dan Duncan Neurological Research Institute, the world's first basic research institute dedicated to childhood neurological diseases. The hospital also followed a growing trend and opened a satellite facility, the Texas Children's West Campus outpatient clinic building, outside the campus of the Texas Medical Center in west Houston.[27]

Among the Texas Medical Center's many great hospitals stands the largest Veterans Administration hospital in the United States, known today as the Michael E. DeBakey Veterans Affairs Medical Center. The hospital had been established as a naval hospital near the end of World War II, but on April 14, 1949, the 500-bed naval hospital facility was transferred to the Veterans Administration and renamed the United States Veterans Administration Hospital. It became a member institution in

1985, and the following year officials held groundbreaking ceremonies to build a new, $246 million replacement facility. The new, state-of-the-art, 1,037-bed facility opened on the same 118-acre site, and the old hospital was later demolished. In December 2003, in recognition of Dr. Michael DeBakey's efforts on behalf of the nation's veterans, President George W. Bush signed a law that formally changed the name of the hospital to the Michael E. DeBakey Veterans Affairs Medical Center (MED-VAMC). Among his many accomplishments, DeBakey had helped to establish the system of treating military personnel returning from the war after World War II, a concept that evolved into the Veterans Health Administration system. Two years later, MEDVAMC opened Fisher House to provide housing and emotional support for families of veterans receiving treatment at the hospital. Fisher House is available free of charge to families of veterans being treated for long-term illnesses.[28]

Over the years, other hospitals opened in or near the Texas Medical Center, including a new Shriners Hospital and the Diagnostic Center Hospital. During the 1990s *U.S. News and World Report* began publishing its annual ratings of US hospitals. From 1990 to the present, several Texas Medical Center institutions have consistently received top rankings, including the M. D. Anderson Cancer Center, the Memorial Hermann Healthcare System, TIRR, St. Luke's Episcopal Hospital, Methodist Hospital, and Texas Children's Hospital.

## Other Institutions

In addition to the hospitals and medical schools, a host of other health-related institutions form this unique conglomeration known as the Texas Medical Center (see appendix 2). Some of these include the City of Houston Department of Health and Human Services, which became a member institution in 1963, and the Gulf Coast Regional Blood Center, established by the Harris County Medical Society in 1975 and dedicated to ensuring a safe, adequate blood supply to Harris County and the surrounding Texas Gulf Coast and East Texas regions. Ronald McDonald House, which first opened in 1981, now has several locations to provide a home for families of children undergoing treatment for cancer and other serious illnesses. The Texas Medical Center has a variety of other nonprofit member institutions, including Houston Hospice, St.

Anthony Center (a geriatric and rehabilitation center), and the YMCA Child Care Center at Texas Medical Center. Over the years, the Houston Academy of Medicine–Texas Medical Center Library has grown in size and reknown, becoming one of the largest medical libraries in the nation and one of eight regional libraries of the National Library of Medicine. In 1983 the Harris County medical examiner's office, the Joseph A. Jachimczyk Forensic Center, became a member institution. The LifeGift Organ Donation Center, which has the primary responsibility of providing organs to the transplant centers of Hermann Hospital, Methodist Hospital, St. Luke's Episcopal Hospital, and Texas Children's Hospital, became a member institution in 1989. And in 1996 the Harris County Medical Society and the Houston Academy of Medicine opened a medical museum known today as the John P. McGovern Museum of Health and Medical Science.

The Texas Medical Center continued to grow even as this manuscript was being completed. On May 14, 2012, the executive committee of the Texas Medical Center's board of directors voted to approve the membership of the Sabin Vaccine Institute, making it the fifty-first member institution of the world's largest medical complex. Headquartered in Washington, DC, and named for oral polio vaccine developer Dr. Albert Sabin, the institute is a nonprofit organization made up of scientists, researchers, and advocates who work to develop new vaccines for diseases that plague the world's poorest people. In September 2011 its vaccine development program relocated to Texas Children's Hospital as a joint program of the Sabin Vaccine Institute, Texas Children's Hospital, and Baylor College of Medicine. Headquarters for the institute's advocacy and education programs remained in Washington, DC. The president of the institute, Peter Hotez, a world-renowned expert on "neglected diseases," spoke about the opportunities the new relationship offered. "This collaboration among institutions represents an extraordinary opportunity to make an important difference in global health," said Hotez. "The Sabin Vaccine Institute is honored to be a member of the Texas Medical Center and looks forward to harnessing the scientific horsepower available here." In addition to his work at the Sabin Vaccine Institute, Hotez is the founding dean of the National School of Tropical Medicine at Baylor College of Medicine, the only school of its kind in the United States.[29]

On June 6, 2012, the Texas Medical Center added a fifty-second institution when the executive committee of the board of directors approved DePelchin Children's Center as the newest member institution. Formerly the DePelchin Faith Home and Children's Bureau, the center was established in 1892 by Kezia Payne DePelchin as a shelter for orphaned children. Today the center provides comprehensive mental health, prevention, and early intervention services for children and adolescents, in addition to its foster care and adoption services, at over sixty locations in Harris, Montgomery, Galveston, Fort Bend, and Waller Counties. "DePelchin Children's Center's mission of strengthening the lives of children by enhancing their mental health and physical well being aligns perfectly with the work being done in the Texas Medical Center on behalf of children," said Texas Medical Center president Richard Wainerdi. "DePelchin's membership in the Texas Medical Center will lead to enhanced collaboration with TMC institutions, which will benefit children, their families and the community."[30]

Although many people and institutions can claim credit for their part in building this amazing medical complex, few would dispute the role of the M. D. Anderson Foundation as the driving force behind it. More than sixty-five years after it was founded, the Texas Medical Center stands as the M. D. Anderson Foundation's greatest achievement. The medical center has continued to grow in its physical size, number of member institutions, patients served, and its renowned position of being home to some of the leading health care institutions in the world. By 2013, it had over fifty member institutions, including three medical schools, six nursing schools, fourteen hospitals, and twenty-one academic institutions. In terms of land, the Texas Medical Center has expanded from the original 134 acres, donated by the M. D. Anderson Foundation, to over 1,300 acres, about the size of the inner loop area of Chicago. Its 280 buildings accommodate approximately 7.1 million patient visits annually and house 92,500 employees, including scientists, researchers, and physicians, about 2,000 of whom are international. On average, about 160,000 people visit the medical center every day. Each year, its educational institutions enroll about 34,000 full-time students and host 7,000 visiting scientists, researchers, and students, including international students. Its hospitals deliver 28,000 babies and perform 350,000 surgeries annually, and there are 6,900 hospital beds and 400 bassinets to accommodate these patients. All in all, the Texas Medical Center has an annual economic impact of some $14 billion on the greater Houston area. And on an annual basis, its institutions spend about $1.8 billion on research and provide $1.2 billion for indigent care.[31]

Just as in the early days, construction continues to be a major characteristic of the Texas Medical Center. The most recent growth spurt added approximately 33 percent to its size, with an additional 10 million square feet of space, some of which will be available for future use. In addition to extending the main campus, many Texas Medical Center institutions have also been expanding into Houston's suburbs and beyond. President and CEO Richard Wainerdi observed that the new wave of expansion marked a change in the concept of the medical center. "When we started, this was a collection of hospitals and schools and institutions. It has now become a collection of systems." Many of the original hospitals, for example, now have multiple locations throughout the greater Houston area and even as far away as other countries. With all of the expansion over the years, Wainerdi stated that the medical center has nevertheless remained true to the ideals of its founders in its efforts to foster collaboration between the institutions: "We keep growing and we keep adding institutions. We want to bring together a lot of collaboration—all of these things can be synergistic. And that is the concept that the M. D. Anderson Foundation and Dr. Bertner and the founders had in mind. The whole concept is that we come together, we live together, and we try to create synergisms that are positive. What has been established here is this asset for the community and for the world. That is why we think this is a great model for the future."[32]

Although much has changed during the more than sixty years of the Texas Medical Center, the spirit that enabled it to achieve its present worldwide prominence continues to flourish. TMC remains an enthusiastic advocate for its member institutions and a watchful guardian of the most unique medical complex in the world. It has also been very effective in its "city hall" functions, continuing to be in the forefront of planning for the future, maintaining architectural standards throughout the campus, and encouraging cooperation on the part of the institutions. TMC installed a geographic information system (GIS) to provide and analyze geographic data for improved planning and also completed

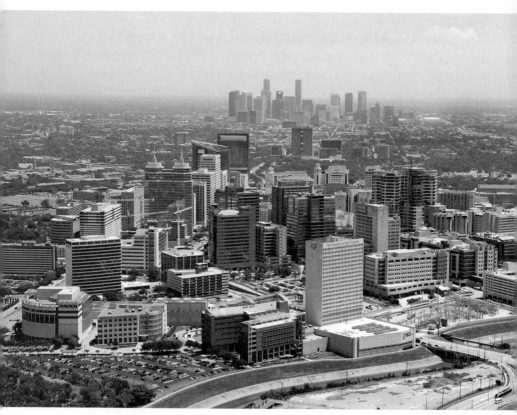

*Looking north over the Texas Medical Center, 2011. Photo by University of Texas Office of Communications; courtesy of Texas Medical Center.*

a $44 million upgrade of utilities and streets to accommodate future growth. The Texas Medical Center has a Mid-Campus and a South Campus to accommodate the continuing need for more space, and its member institutions have spread out as well. Among these is UTMB in Galveston and its health clinics in Friendswood, League City, Texas City, Dickinson, Nassau Bay, and Webster. In addition, many of the medical center's hospitals have opened satellite clinics, and facilities have spread all across the greater Houston area and, as mentioned above, reach out around the world. Currently, with twenty-seven agencies of government and twenty-seven private, not-for-profit institutions, the Texas Medical Center has become the "city of health" that its founders envisioned, but in a more spectacular manner than they might have imagined. "All these institutions are proud of being part of something that includes reputable and important colleagues. That means something to them," said Richard Wainerdi.[33]

The Texas Medical Center is unique in medical history and remains a very special place to the thousands of people who have labored in its many institutions and to the multitude of patients whose lives have been touched by the incredible work of these medical professionals over the years. "We have changed the lives of people for a very long time," said Wainerdi. Calling the Texas Medical Center "a place of magic," Wainerdi attributes its success to the "tens of thousands of dedicated people like Dr. Michael DeBakey, Dr. Denton Cooley, Dr. Ralph Feigin, and thousands more whose names are not recorded." Before Wainerdi retired on January 1, 2013, he acknowledged the many challenges ahead for his successor, Dr. Robert C. Robbins. But the Texas Medical Center continues to enjoy support from the people of greater Houston, the state of Texas, and the many philanthropic foundations that have provided funds throughout its history. As the medical center continues to fulfill its mission of promoting the "highest quality health status for all people" and encouraging its member institutions in their quest to achieve "the highest possible standards of patient and preventive care, of research and education, and of local, national, and international community well being," it also carries on the bold objectives of its founders and the noble principles of its major benefactor, Monroe Dunaway Anderson. When talking about the impact of the Texas Medical Center, Wainerdi often quotes former first lady Barbara Bush, who reportedly said, "The Texas Medical Center is Houston's gift to the world." One might add that the origins of that "gift to the world" are found in Monroe D. Anderson's gift to the people of Houston when, on July 9, 1936, he signed a trust indenture and created the M. D. Anderson Foundation. How wonderfully ironic, then, that the legacy of this quiet, soft-spoken man from Jackson, Tennessee, a man who shunned the spotlight during his lifetime, continues to touch so many people in such good ways all around the world.[34]

# Epilogue

## The Enduring Legacy
## of Monroe Dunaway Anderson

During the years since it was created in 1936, the M. D. Anderson Foundation has given millions of dollars to a wide variety of educational, charitable, and health-related institutions, all part of the exceptional legacy of Monroe Dunaway Anderson. Although this book focused on the Texas Medical Center and the Anderson Foundation's role in its creation, it is useful here to summarize the continuing philanthropic work of the foundation and the subsequent developments related to the city of Houston, Anderson, Clayton & Company, and Fulbright, Crooker, Freeman & Bates, all of which had a significant part in the history of the foundation.

One of the key factors in the story of the M. D. Anderson Foundation has been its location in Houston. As the city grew to maturity during the twentieth century, Houston continued to be a business-friendly, fertile environment in which entrepreneurs launched homegrown businesses and countless firms such as Anderson, Clayton & Company established themselves as industry leaders. Their success made many of these business leaders very wealthy, and this, in turn, often motivated a sense of obligation and a desire to give something back to the community in which they had achieved so much. Although this is generally true in most communities, this altruism and beneficence seemed especially dominant in Houston. One observer noted that, "they *believed* in philanthropy. They not only believed in philanthropy, but if you did not contribute to the cultural life of Houston, you were a poor citizen."

It may be, in part, that Houston is a young city by comparison, and succeeding business leaders felt strongly that they wanted to build it into something better for themselves and succeeding generations. George H. Hermann, Robert A. Welch, Jesse H. Jones, Hugh Roy Cullen, Will and Ben Clayton, Herman and George Brown, and, of course, Monroe D. Anderson are but a few of the city's early benefactors who recognized the important part the city had in their success and established philanthropic foundations as a means of giving back to the community.

At the time that the Anderson trustees formally established the Texas Medical Center in 1945, Houston was in the midst of an economic expansion that began before World War II, and its population had grown accordingly, to about 448,000. By 1962, the end of the medical center's founding era, Houston's population had increased dramatically to 1,091,800, making it the sixth-largest city in the United States. Houston was home to the third-largest seaport in the nation, handling some fifty-nine million tons of cargo annually, and was first in refineries, pipeline transmission, and the manufacture of petroleum equipment. During the next fifty years Houston endured its share of adversity and prosperity, but its "can do" spirit remained undaunted, and the city continued to attract new businesses, from small entrepreneurs to Fortune 500 companies, and even became home to the NASA Manned Space Center, later renamed the Johnson Space Center. By the 1980s, energy businesses dominated Houston's economy, with about 85 percent of all jobs in the energy-related fields, giving rise to the slogan "Energy Capital of the World." Although Houston today remains the home of some 5,000 energy-related firms, after surviving the economic crash of the mid-1980s, the overall economy is now more diverse, with many jobs being developed in nonenergy areas such as medicine, aerospace, manufacturing, technology, and services. The Port of Houston continues to be one of the main drivers of the city's economic growth and in 2012 was ranked first in the nation in international tonnage, first in imports to the United States, second in total tonnage handled, and the tenth-largest port in the world. In addition, Houston is home to a $15 billion petrochemical complex, the largest in the nation and second-largest in the world. Thus, all of the features that initially attracted Anderson, Clayton & Company to Houston early in the twentieth century continue to attract businesses and entrepreneurs to the city today.[1]

Although Houston has continued to thrive, albeit with its share of setbacks and challenges along the way, the same cannot be said for Anderson, Clayton, & Company, the firm that built the fortune on which the M. D. Anderson Foundation was established. By the end of World War II, Anderson, Clayton had become the largest cotton-trading firm in the world. During the postwar years, the firm, generally known as ACCO, diversified into industrial production, government warehousing services, and a foods division that included Chiffon margarine and Seven Seas salad dressing. By the mid-1960s ACCO was invested in major publicly traded companies in Mexico and Brazil, including cotton-related operations and coffee, cocoa, and soybean processing, in addition to its integrated worldwide cotton operations. The cotton industry, however, had changed, and new government regulations made it increasingly difficult for the company's US cotton operations to remain profitable. Consequently, during the 1960s, the firm began to divest most of its cotton businesses, at least in the United States, and to focus on other areas related mainly to food products. By the early 1970s, ACCO had ceased nearly all of its cotton merchandising except in Mexico and Brazil. Soon the firm was a major player in the insurance industry through its acquisition of Ranger Insurance and, later, American Founders Life Insurance Company. It also acquired Igloo Corporation (a producer of thermoplastic beverage containers and ice chests) and Gaines Pet Foods Company and eventually employed approximately 25,000 people worldwide in its many divisions.[2]

During the mid-1980s, shortly after ACCO acquired Gaines, the company's executives saw a need to make major changes if the firm was to maximize its value to its stockholders. With all of its diversity, stockbrokers could not easily determine whether ACCO was primarily a trading company, a food company, or an insurance business. This confusion kept the price of the company's stock very low. As the firm's former vice president, Merrill Glasgow, recalled, "Anderson Clayton was not an attractive investment or acquisition target for anybody because there were just too many different odds and ends. They all were making money, but in terms of an acquisition, it was not a package you wanted to buy." When stockholders sold shares in the company, they sold at a very low price-to-earnings ratio because analysts did not understand the stock. In order to maximize the value of its stock, the company needed to make major changes, so the directors began to consider several options.[3]

Initially, one plan had been to take the company private through an employee stock ownership plan. But at about the same time, because the company was undervalued with the parts worth more than the whole and because of the profitability of the Gaines Pet Foods division, ACCO suddenly became an attractive acquisition target. Ultimately, with eyes primarily on the Gaines division, both Quaker Oats and Ralston Purina began efforts to acquire the company. Pet foods were a major part of their respective businesses, and both firms wanted to add the Gaines brand to their holdings. After a fierce bidding war, Quaker Oats submitted the highest bid, and on September 27, 1986, the ACCO board announced it had agreed to sell the firm to Quaker Oats for $66 per share, or about $810 million total. Two years earlier the stock had been trading at $32 per share.[4]

The sale meant the end of Anderson, Clayton & Company, but it worked out well for the great majority of employees and all stockholders. Former ACCO executive vice president John Fichter later summarized the company's history, noting that it was like "a Harvard Business School case of how some really high-quality people created a small company and then had the vision and the courage to build it into a large, international business." But despite its corporate demise, the legacy of Anderson, Clayton & Company continues in the form of numerous charitable foundations established by the company's founders and their successors. One of the most significant, however, is the M. D. Anderson Foundation. Thus, the impact of a small cotton-trading firm established in 1904 continues into the present because of the success of that company and the civic-mindedness of Monroe D. Anderson. "You can trace it all the way back to him," said attorney Gibson Gayle Jr., longtime trustee and former president (1990–2010) of the M. D. Anderson Foundation.[5]

Monroe Anderson was both a banker and an entrepreneur, characteristics that also made him a person of vision with an extremely practical bent. His friends knew him as a man with a strong sense of compassion and a willingness to help those in need who either could not help themselves or who were struggling hard to improve their own lives. Both frugal and generous, Anderson deeply desired to help the working classes, the sick and aged, and those striving to improve the human condition through "health, science, education, and advancement and diffusion of knowledge and understanding among the people," but he had little patience for the slothful or profligate. Anderson had a keen eye for recognizing character in people and surrounded himself with ambitious, talented men of integrity. One of the first in this circle was the young attorney Clarence Fulbright, whom Anderson and Will Clayton convinced to open his own office and take on some of the legal affairs of Anderson, Clayton & Company. In time, two of the men who became partners in Fulbright's law firm—William B. Bates and John H. Freeman—also became close friends, confidants, and the men Anderson entrusted with helping him create and run his foundation.[6]

Although they did not have a specific plan for the foundation when Anderson died in 1939, Freeman and Bates had a good sense of what Anderson would have wanted to do. When the opportunity arose for the foundation to take a leading role in creating a new medical center, the trustees boldly seized the initiative, and the Anderson Foundation became the driving force behind the founding of what many imagined as a "city of health" in Houston. As plans for the medical center began to evolve, it was not only the funding that was important, but also the trustees' wisdom, leadership, and ability to gain the support of the broader community that helped move events forward. Freeman, Bates, and later Horace M. Wilkins made crucial decisions at key moments, all having a long-term impact on the development of the Texas Medical Center. Thus, the largest medical complex in the world today is also one of the most innovative. It is not owned or managed by one entity but is a collection of independent, nonprofit institutions dedicated to medical research, education, and patient care. Although at times this arrangement has been a little disorderly, the positive impact of this organizational structure, put in place by the trustees of the Anderson Foundation when they established the medical center, has provided a setting in which each member institution could develop and thrive on its own and yet still be part of something unique in medical history.

The law firm that helped Monroe Anderson create his charitable foundation, Fulbright, Crooker & Freeman, continued as Fulbright & Jaworski LLP, one of the largest law firms in the United States. In November 2012 Fulbright & Jaworski announced that it would merge with the London-based firm Norton Rose, effective June 2013. Fulbright & Jaworski had grown into a full-service international law firm that employed about 900 lawyers in seventeen offices around the world, including London, Munich, Dubai, Riyadh, Hong Kong, and Beijing. The new firm would be known as Norton Rose Fulbright and would have some 3,800 lawyers in fifty-five offices around the world, making it one of the ten largest global legal practices. Lawyers from Fulbright & Jaworski have served on the board of trustees of the M. D. Anderson Foundation throughout its history and have provided legal services for the Texas Medical Center and many of its institutions from the beginning. One of the reasons for the success of this relationship between the Anderson Foundation and the Fulbright attorneys has been the deep sense of obligation on the part of the attorneys to what they have always viewed as a sacred trust from Monroe Anderson. "No question about it," stated Gibson Gayle, who is also a former managing partner of Fulbright & Jaworski. "And he made it very clear to Freeman and Bates during the last years of his life that he was looking to them and their successor trustees to see that that foundation was run with honor, dignity, and with total integrity. The responsibility was put on this law firm by Monroe D. Anderson. I have no doubt about that." In fact, throughout its history, the M. D. Anderson Foundation has had only a small number of trustees, all of whom served capably, generally for fairly long periods of time (see appendix 1). The law firm first established by Clarence Fulbright and John Crooker continues to provide three of the four trustees to each board and also handles the foundation's legal services, exactly as Monroe Anderson intended. In 1957 the board added a fourth position with the appointment of Leon Jaworski, who joined trustees William B. Bates, John H. Freeman, and Warren S. Bellows. Since then, only eight other men have served on the board of trustees: A. G. McNeese, Hugh Q. Buck, Gibson Gayle Jr., Kraft W. Eidman, Charles W. Hall, Uriel E. Dutton, Jack T. Trotter, and Leo E. Linbeck Jr.[7]

The two last surviving members of the foundation's original board of trustees, William B. Bates and John H. Freeman, both remained on the board into their advanced years. Bates died in Houston on April 17, 1974, at age eighty-five. In addition to being one of the founders of the Anderson Foundation and the Texas Medical Center, Bates was instrumental in establishing the University of Houston as a four-year

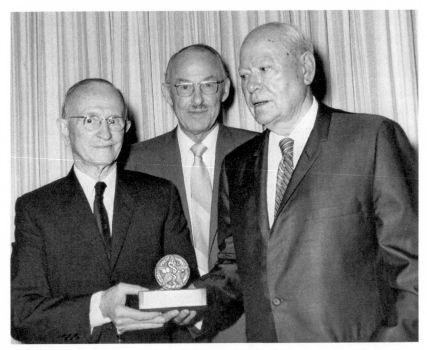

*Frederick C. Elliott, R. Lee Clark, and William B. Bates at a ceremony in 1970 honoring Elliott and Bates for their contributions as founders of the Texas Medical Center. Courtesy of John P. McGovern Historical Collections and Research Center, Texas Medical Center Library.*

institution. He served as vice chairman of the original board of regents and as chairman following the death of Hugh Roy Cullen in 1957. He continued to serve as a regent after the university became a state institution, from 1963 until 1971. Bates was also deeply involved in the San Jacinto Monument and museum. After funeral services in Houston, he was buried at the Nacogdoches Oak Grove Cemetery, in his beloved East Texas. University of Houston president Philip G. Hoffman paid tribute to Bates, saying, "He will be remembered as long as there is a Houston, or an expanding city to which men of Colonel Bates's high level of ability and commitment are drawn for their life work." And Newton Gresham, a partner in the Fulbright firm, in a statement for the Philosophical Society of Texas, wrote, "William Bartholomew Bates was truly a giant in this earth, a man of quiet power, a true friend and an exemplar of the good and true husband and father. For all of these qualities and for his many works, he should and will be remembered."[8]

Six years later, on Sunday, July 13, 1980, ninety-three-year-old John H. Freeman died at his home in Houston. After funeral services the following Wednesday, he was buried at Houston's Glenwood Cemetery. During his lifetime Freeman was highly regarded as an attorney, widely recognized for his role in establishing the Texas Medical Center, and greatly admired for his remarkable humility. He was known to keep a plaque in his office that stated, "There is no limit to what a man can do if he does not care who gets the credit." Freeman served as president of the M. D. Anderson Foundation from 1949 to 1976 and was a trustee for forty-four years. Months before he died, the *Houston Post* honored Freeman in an editorial, saying in part, "Few men have done as much for their community as John Freeman. Perhaps more important, in the lengthening history of Houston, he has given to succeeding generations of community leaders an example and an ideal. . . . John Freeman's greatness has a rare purity." Freeman's friend and colleague, attorney Leon Jaworski, observed, "What makes our world so great is individuals like him. He was a great man and one of the most interesting men I ever knew. But you'd never hear him talk about himself."[9]

Years later Gibson Gayle reflected on the role of the Anderson Foundation and its original trustees in creating the Texas Medical Center. "The credit goes to Mr. Anderson for setting it up and providing the money," said Gayle, "and then to Freeman and Bates primarily for putting through whatever had to be done to create the Texas Medical Center. They are the men that put it together." Author N. Don Macon, who conducted a series of videotaped oral history interviews with many of the medical center's founders during the 1970s, later wrote about the crucial role of the Anderson Foundation's early trustees. "The medical center idea may have been dreamed of by a number of men in one form or another," stated Macon. "But the idea was brought to reality principally by the trustees of the M. D. Anderson Foundation. Events of the moment played a great part in getting the center underway. But the endless day-to-day details, the careful planning, the wholesome involvement of the community, were worked out by the trustees of the Anderson Foundation—Colonel Bates, John Freeman, and Horace Wilkins."[10]

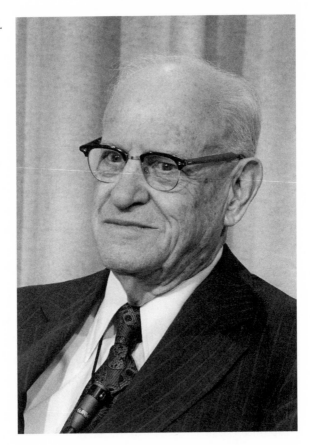

*John H. Freeman, 1978.*
*Courtesy of Fulbright*
*& Jaworski LLP.*

It is interesting to note that the M. D. Anderson Foundation continues to reflect the character of its founding benefactor, Monroe Dunaway Anderson, a man who preferred to work in the background and shunned publicity. So too has his foundation operated over the years. The trustees quietly have gone about the work of managing the foundation's assets and distributing grants in the manner prescribed by the original trust indenture. But this low-key approach is not to say that the M. D. Anderson Foundation has not had a substantial impact. During the years since Monroe Anderson established his foundation, the succeeding trustees have managed the assets with great care and skill. Thus, the original corpus of $19 million grew to about $150 million before the economic crisis of 2008. Across the country, investors at every level, including charitable foundations, suffered significant setbacks to their portfolios during the recession. But with the economy recovering by the end of 2011, the Anderson Foundation was on the rebound. After starting out with $19 million from Monroe Anderson's estate, it is estimated that during its first seventy-five years, the foundation has given away over $276 million.

Over the years, as Gibson Gayle noted, "the biggest thing in the history of the foundation was the donation of the land to the Texas Medical Center." In addition to this early, crucial support, the Anderson Foundation has continued to give to the cancer hospital, now known as the M. D. Anderson Cancer Center, and to Baylor College of Medicine, Memorial Hermann Hospital, Methodist Hospital, St. Luke's Episcopal Hospital, Texas Children's Hospital, Texas Woman's University, and almost every private entity in the medical center. Attorney Charles W. Hall, who became president of the Anderson Foundation in 2010, described its continuing role in the world of Houston's philanthropic foundations, stating, "The Anderson Foundation is a large, 'small foundation.' We support various organizations, mostly in Houston, and mostly connected to the Medical Center." The Anderson Foundation has been a primary financial supporter throughout the years, donating an estimated $81 million to the Texas Medical Center and its member institutions, including approximately $41.3 million to the medical and nursing schools, and some $13.3 million to the medical center's hospitals. These grants, in turn, have had a multiplier effect, fostering matching funds from government agencies, other private philanthropic foundations, and individual and corporate donors. Dr. Richard E. Wainerdi, president of the Texas Medical Center until his retirement at the beginning of 2013, summarized the importance of the M. D. Anderson Foundation, noting, "They have been, through the years, one of the major supporters of the Texas Medical Center itself—very generous in terms of their philanthropic support but also in terms of the support of their trustees who have been on our board."[11]

The impact of private philanthropy, and particularly the M. D. Anderson Foundation, has been crucial to the development of the Texas Medical Center. David Underwood, chairman of the board of the Medical Center, stated, "Were it not for philanthropy, the Texas Medical Center would not exist. Were it not for Monroe Dunaway Anderson and his legacy and his Foundation, and were it not for John Freeman and Dr.

Bertner and Colonel Bates buying the concept of a city of medicine, it simply would not exist as it is today. It is a remarkable story [and] it starts with philanthropy." Although the Anderson Foundation was the catalyst in launching the Texas Medical Center, it is important to note that many other philanthropies and private donors have contributed as well, a list that includes familiar names in Houston's business history, much too extensive to include here but indispensable nevertheless.[12]

In addition to its many grants to the Texas Medical Center over the years, the M. D. Anderson Foundation has provided over $63 million to schools and educational programs, with about $43 million going to institutions of higher education, apart from what the foundation has donated to medical schools. The Anderson Foundation also has provided support to the Houston Ballet, Houston Grand Opera, Houston Symphony, the Museum of Fine Arts, Houston, the YMCA, historical societies and museums, the Red Cross, and a host of other charitable organizations, mainly in the greater Houston area but also in other places in Texas and across the country.

In 2002 the foundation's trustees discovered a potential conflict between the state laws under which the foundation was originally established as a common law charitable trust in 1936 and current federal laws regarding distribution of funds. Under the original charter, only money earned from the corpus of the foundation could be given away in grants. The principal was to be left untouched so it could continue to earn from investments and provide a source for funds in perpetuity. But the federal tax laws regarding distributions and other activities of tax-exempt private foundations had developed to the degree that the trustees saw a need to modernize the governance of the foundation to be more easily in compliance. The federal law required that 5 percent of the market value of the foundation during the previous year had to be distributed in grants. Eager to avoid any complications related to the foundation, the trustees engaged the help of outside counsel and changed the way it was organized, from a charitable trust to a charitable corporation. The new organizational structure included a provision that, in order to comply with the law, if the trustees had to make some part of the distributions out of the principal, they could do so and still be in compliance with both the state and federal regulations. By changing from a common law trust to a Texas nonprofit corporation, the foundation adopted more flexible and modern legal guidelines from which to operate. The Anderson Foundation's new status as a charitable or nonprofit corporation ensured that it could continue its philanthropic work and meet the requirements of both the State of Texas and federal laws.[13]

Throughout the years, then, the men who succeeded Bates, Freeman, and Wilkins as trustees of the Anderson Foundation remained steadfast in adhering to the original mission and following the philanthropic principles that Monroe D. Anderson outlined before his death. Interestingly, it is not uncommon for succeeding boards to veer away from the founding grantor's wishes in managing philanthropic foundations. By contrast, the trustees of the M. D. Anderson Foundation faithfully followed Anderson's stated wishes and made it possible for this "large, small foundation" to have a profound impact, not only in Houston but in Texas and beyond, in part through its continuing support of the Texas Medical Center. "Their role continues," said Richard Wainerdi. "First, [the Anderson Foundation] gave birth to the Texas Medical Center. And through the years, because of the consistency of the trustees, their relationship to us has been very positive and they have helped, as individuals, in keeping the flame going. I think it cannot be overemphasized how important they are. I would call them the patrons of the Texas Medical Center."[14]

The work of the M. D. Anderson Foundation continues today, the enduring legacy of Monroe D. Anderson. Hundreds of organizations, both large and small, have been the beneficiaries of Anderson's desire to give back to his adopted hometown. More importantly, through his foundation, Anderson has touched the lives of thousands of people who have come to the Texas Medical Center either as patients or to work as physicians, nurses, researchers, educators, or staff in its growing list of member institutions. The legacy of M. D. Anderson is manifest every day in the gleaming structures of the Texas Medical Center, in the world-renowned cancer center that bears his name, and in the hundreds of organizations that have been the beneficiaries of his foresight and civic generosity.

Although he did not know it at the time, when Anderson created his charitable foundation in 1936, he also lit a flame that his trustees have kept burning ever since, a flame that shines bright as a beacon of hope to those who are suffering and as an inspiration to the many who have joined the crusade to build the largest place of healing in the world, the Texas Medical Center. Ironically, the man who contributed so much to creating and building this "city of health" did not live long enough to see it or even to know about it. But the men to whom he entrusted his fortune and his foundation proved themselves worthy of their charge. So too have their successors on the Anderson Foundation's board of trustees. And thus today, if one should gaze out upon the great expanse of the world's largest medical center and take a few moments to contemplate the good work that has been accomplished over time in this place of healing, one might recall the epitaph in St. Paul's Cathedral written for the renowned English architect Sir Christopher Wren as also being a fitting memorial for Monroe Dunaway Anderson: ". . . if you seek his monument, look around you."

# Appendix 1

## M. D. Anderson Foundation Trustees, 1936–2013

Monroe D. Anderson . . . . . . . . . . . . . . . . . . . . . . . . . . . . . . . . . . . . .1936–39
William B. Bates* . . . . . . . . . . . . . . . . . . . . . . . . . . . . . . . . . . . . . . .1936–74
Warren S. Bellows . . . . . . . . . . . . . . . . . . . . . . . . . . . . . . . . . . . . . .1953–67
Hugh Q. Buck* . . . . . . . . . . . . . . . . . . . . . . . . . . . . . . . . . . . . . . . . 1974–86
James W. Crownover . . . . . . . . . . . . . . . . . . . . . . . . . . . . . . . . . 2013–
Uriel E. Dutton* . . . . . . . . . . . . . . . . . . . . . . . . . . . . . . . . . . . . . . . 1986–
Kraft W. Eidman* . . . . . . . . . . . . . . . . . . . . . . . . . . . . . . . . . . . . . . 1982–86
John H. Freeman* . . . . . . . . . . . . . . . . . . . . . . . . . . . . . . . . . . . . . . 1936–80
Gibson Gayle Jr.* . . . . . . . . . . . . . . . . . . . . . . . . . . . . . . . . . . . . . . 1980–
Charles W. Hall* . . . . . . . . . . . . . . . . . . . . . . . . . . . . . . . . . . . . . . . 1986–
Leon Jaworski* . . . . . . . . . . . . . . . . . . . . . . . . . . . . . . . . . . . . . . . . 1957–82
Leo S. Linbeck Jr. . . . . . . . . . . . . . . . . . . . . . . . . . . . . . . . . . . . . . . 2010–13
A. G. McNeese Jr. . . . . . . . . . . . . . . . . . . . . . . . . . . . . . . . . . . . . . . 1967–90
Jack T. Trotter . . . . . . . . . . . . . . . . . . . . . . . . . . . . . . . . . . . . . 1991–2009
Horace M. Wilkins . . . . . . . . . . . . . . . . . . . . . . . . . . . . . . . . . . . . . 1940–53

*Trustees affiliated with Fulbright & Jaworski LLP and its predecessors

# Appendix 2

## Texas Medical Center Member Institutions

Baylor College of Medicine (1943)
Children's Memorial Hermann Hospital (1986)
City of Houston Department of Health and Human Services (1963)
DePelchin Children's Center (2012)
Gulf Coast Regional Blood Center (1988)
Harris County Hospital District–Ben Taub General Hospital (1960)
Harris County Hospital District–Lyndon B. Johnson General Hospital (1989)
Harris County Hospital District–Quentin Mease Community Hospital (1986)
Harris County Medical Society (1954)
Harris County Public Health and Environmental Services (2007)
Houston Academy of Medicine (1952)
Houston Academy of Medicine–Texas Medical Center Library (1949)
Houston Community College System (1977)
Houston Hospice (1983)
Institute of Religion (1955)
John P. McGovern Museum of Health and Medical Science (1995)
Joseph A. Jachimczyk Forensic Center (1983)
LifeGift Organ Donation Center (1989)
Memorial Hermann–Texas Medical Center (1944)
Menninger Clinic (2012)
Methodist Hospital (1950)
Michael E. DeBakey High School for Health Professions (1973)
Michael E. DeBakey Veterans Affairs Medical Center–Houston (1985)
Prairie View A&M University College of Nursing (1982)

Rice University (2003)

Ronald McDonald House Houston (1989)

Sabin Vaccine Institute (2012)

St. Dominic Village (2008)

St. Luke's Episcopal Health System (1951)

Shriners Hospitals for Children–Houston (1952)

Shriners Hospitals for Children–Galveston (2011)

Texas A&M University Health Science Center–Houston (1986)

Texas Children's Hospital (1951)

Texas Heart Institute (1971)

Texas Medical Center (1945)

Texas Medical Center Hospital Laundry Cooperative Association (1972)

Texas Southern University College of Pharmacy and Health Sciences (2002)

Texas Woman's University Institute of Health Sciences–Houston (1961)

Thermal Energy Corporation (TECO; 1978)

TIRR Memorial Hermann (Institute for Rehabilitation and Research; 1957)

University of Houston (2009)

University of Houston College of Pharmacy (1980)

University of Houston–Victoria School of Nursing (2012)

University of Texas M. D. Anderson Cancer Center (1942)

University of Texas Medical Branch at Galveston (2010)

University of Texas Health Science Center at Houston (UTHealth; 1972)

University of Texas Health Science Center at Houston School of Dentistry at Houston (1943)

University of Texas Health Science Center at Houston School of Biomedical Sciences at Houston (1970)

University of Texas Health Science Center at Houston Harris County Psychiatric Center (1984)

University of Texas Health Science Center at Houston Brown Foundation Institute of Molecular Medicine for the Prevention of Human Diseases (1995)

University of Texas Medical School at Houston (1971)

University of Texas Health Science Center at Houston School of Biomedical Informatics at Houston (1997)

University of Texas Health Science Center at Houston School of Nursing (1972)
University of Texas Health Science Center at Houston School of Public Health (1970)
Texas Medical Center YMCA (1988)

# *Notes*

## Introduction

1. Marilyn McAdams Sibley, *The Port of Houston: A History* (Austin: University of Texas Press, 1968) 134–38; Joseph Pratt, "8F and Many More: Business and Civic Leadership in Modern Houston," *Houston Review of History and Culture* 1, no. 2 (Summer 2004): 2–6.

2. David Underwood, interview by William H. Kellar, April 20, 2012; Richard E. Wainerdi, interview by William H. Kellar, May 10, 2012.

## Chapter 1

1. Marilyn McAdams Sibley, *The Port of Houston: A History* (Austin: University of Texas Press, 1968), 33–34; Houston History, "Augustus Allen," http://www.houstonhistory.com/citizens/houstonians/history8a.htm (accessed May 9, 2011).

2. Charles H. McCollum, "Surgeons and the Texas Revolution," in *The History of Surgery in Houston: Fifty-Year Anniversary of the Houston Surgical Society,* edited by Kenneth L. Maddox (Austin: Eakin Press, 1998), 3–10, 13–14.

3. Harris County Medical Society, *A History of Organized Medicine in Harris County, Texas* (Houston, 1948), 4; Walter H. Moursund, *Medicine in Greater Houston, 1836–1956,* edited by Mildred Moursund Essig (Houston: Baylor College of Medicine, 1958), 472. Among the new generation of physicians were Drs. S. O. Young Sr., W. D. Robinson, William McCraven, William H. Howard, and L. A. Bryan.

4. Moursund, *Medicine in Greater Houston,* 473.

5. Ibid., 475; "Health of Houston," *Morning Star,* August 29, 1843; Laurens R. Pickard, "Surgery in Houston between the Texas Revolution and 1900," in Maddox, ed. *History of Surgery in Houston,* 16. Yellow fever epidemics struck Houston in 1847, 1853, 1858, 1859, 1863, and 1867.

6. *Telegraph and Texas Register,* August 30, 1836; Houston History, "Our Legacy," http://www.houstonhistory.com/legacy/history6d.htm (accessed October 13, 2010); Marguerite Johnston, *Houston: The Unknown City, 1836–1946* (College Station: Texas A&M University Press, 1991), 46; Sibley, *Port of Houston,* 75. Conversion to 2011 dollars is from http://www.measuringworth.com/uscompare/ (accessed September 6, 2012).

7. Max H. Jacobs and H. Dick Golding, *Houston and Cotton* (Houston: Max H. Jacobs Agency, 1949), 15.

8. Johnston, *Houston,* 22, 53; David G. McComb, *Houston: The Bayou City* (Austin: University of Texas Press, 1970), 19; Find a Grave, "Thomas W. House," http://

www.findagrave.com/cgi-bin/fg.cgi?page=gr&GRid=8477706 (accessed July 12, 2010).

9. Andrew Morrison, *The City of Houston and the State of Texas*, American Cities series (Houston: Geo. W. Englehart, 1891), 75–76.

10. Sibley, *Port of Houston*, 61.

11. Harris County Historical Society, *Houston: A History & Guide* (Houston: Anson Jones Press, 1942), 259; Richard G. Boehm, *Exporting Cotton in Texas: Relationships of Ports and Inland Supply Points* (Austin: University of Texas Press, 1975), 9; Sibley, *Port of Houston*, 58–59, 70.

12. Harris County Historical Society, *Houston*, 68–69; Hugh Hemphill, *The Railroads of San Antonio and South Central Texas* (San Antonio: Maverick Publishing, 2006), 1, 6–7.

13. Joseph A. Pratt, *The Growth of a Refining Region* (Greenwich, Conn.: Jai Press, 1980), 28; Boehm, *Exporting Cotton in Texas*, 4; Jacobs and Golding, *Houston and Cotton*, 15; Sibley, *Port of Houston*, 60–61; Harris County Historical Society, *Houston*, 68.

14. George C. Werner, "Buffalo Bayou, Brazos and Colorado Railway," *Handbook of Texas Online*, http://www.tshaonline.org/handbook/online/articles/BB/eqb16. html (accessed July 30, 2010); Sibley, *Port of Houston*, 74; Pratt, *Growth of a Refining Region*, 2, 15, 23; Walter J. Buenger and Joseph A. Pratt, *But Also Good Business: Texas Commerce Banks and the Financing of Houston and Texas, 1886–1986* (College Station: Texas A&M University Press, 1986), 13, 20–21; Harris County Historical Society, *Houston*, 143.

15. Sibley, *Port of Houston*, 97.

16. Ibid., 69–70, 77.

17. Jacobs and Golding, *Houston and Cotton*, 23; Sibley, *Port of Houston*, 82–83, 87; Marguerite Johnston, *Houston*, 73.

18. Sibley, *Port of Houston*, 112, 120.

19. Buenger and Pratt, *But Also Good Business*, 27; Sibley, *Port of Houston*, 97.

20. Charles F. Morse, *City of Houston and Harris County: World's Columbian Exposition Souvenir–1893* (Washington, DC: Library of Congress, 1893), 33; Jacobs and Golding, *Houston and Cotton*, 25–27.

21. Pratt, *Growth of a Refining Region*, 19; Harris County Historical Society, *Houston*, 102.

22. Harris County Medical Society, *History of Organized Medicine in Harris County*, 5, 8, 10–14; Harris County Medical Society, "History of HCMS," http://www.hcms. org/Template.aspx?id=53 (accessed April 16, 2011). By 1912, the Harris County Medical Society had grown to 133 members; it reached 519 in 1940. In 2011 the organization had more than 9,000 members.

23. Pickard, "Surgery in Houston," 19–20.

24. Ibid.; Moursund, *Medicine in Greater Houston*, 475.

25. Moursund, 289–92; Johnston, *Houston,* 58, 96; Chester R. Burns, *Saving Lives, Training Caregivers, Making Discoveries: A Centennial History of the University of Texas Medical Branch at Galveston* (Austin: Texas State Historical Association, 2003), 9–10. The Sisters of Charity of the Incarnate Word established St. Mary's Infirmary in Galveston in 1876. It expanded over the years, and by 1887 St. Mary's Infirmary had grown to a three-story, 250-bed hospital.

26. Moursund, *Medicine in Greater Houston,* 281–85.

27. Ibid., 293–99; Marilyn McAdams Sibley, *The Methodist Hospital of Houston: Serving the World* (Austin: Texas State Historical Association, 1989), 9–11; Betty Chapman, "Nursing Profession Embarked on Mission of Mercy 100 Years Ago," *Houston Business Journal,* May 5, 2000, reprinted July 22, 2011.

28. Moursund, *Medicine in Greater Houston,* 300–301.

29. In addition to the hospitals within the city limits of Houston, physicians in the area known as Houston Heights were also very active in their efforts to provide hospital care and attempted to open several facilities in the community. Among the best known were the Texas Christian Sanitarium, which opened in 1908 in the old Houston Heights Hotel building, and the Heights Clinic Hospital, which opened at 1919 Ashland Avenue in 1923. Within a few years, the Texas Christian Sanitarium closed, and in February 1912 the building became the Heights Sanitarium, serving as a home for "feeble-minded" patients. The staff focused on providing care for the mentally ill and treating drug and alcohol addictions until a fire on June 1, 1915, destroyed the old structure. One of the final additions in the Heights, the Heights Clinic Hospital, was established by Dr. Thomas A. Sinclair, who had been the house physician at the Texas Christian Sanitarium, and Dr. Mylie Durham Sr. The modest six-bed hospital proved to be a successful endeavor. It offered emergency care and soon expanded to forty-five beds. In 1940 the hospital underwent a full renovation and ultimately added a maternity wing in 1954. Mylie Durham had two sons who followed him into medicine. Dr. Mylie Durham Jr. entered family practice, and Dr. Charles Durham specialized in obstetrics and gynecology. See Moursund, *Medicine in Greater Houston,* 281–88; Flora L. Roeder and Richard J. Andrassy, "Surgery in Houston between 1900 and 1940," in Maddox, ed., *History of Surgery in Houston,* 22; Sister M. Agatha, *The History of Houston Heights, 1891–1918* (Houston: Premier Printing, 1956), 49–51.

30. Moursund, *Medicine in Greater Houston,* 286–88. In 1938 a new eleven-story, 500-bed Jefferson Davis Hospital was constructed just west of downtown on Allen Parkway. Initially the hospital had no intensive care units; patients were treated in open wards. The trauma center consisted of one shock room, two treatment rooms, and two holding areas. Harris Health System, "A Proud History of Caring," https://www.harrishealth.org/en/about-us/who-we-are/pages/history.aspx (accessed July 28, 2013); Riverside General Hospital, "Riverside General Hospital History," http://

www.riversidegeneralhospital.org/getpage.php?name=houston&sub=About%20Us (accessed October 17, 2011).

31. Moursund, *Medicine in Greater Houston,* 479–81.

32. Ibid., 482–83. According to Moursund, in 1911 the City Health Department included Dr. F. J. Slataper, the city pathologist in charge of the health laboratory; Dr. W. W. Ralston, school medical inspector; and Dr. George W. Larendon, city health officer. The Board of Health was composed of Drs. Joe Stuart, president, W. A. Archer, J. W. Scott, Sidney J. Smith, J. D. Duckett, and S. H. Hillen.

33. Jacobs and Golding, *Houston and Cotton,* 25; Buenger and Pratt, *But Also Good Business,* 23.

34. Harris County Historical Society, *Houston,* 108–109, 112–14, 156; Sibley, *Port of Houston,* 147, 160.

35. Joe R. Feagin, *Free Enterprise City: Houston in Political-Economic Perspective* (New Brunswick, N.J.: Rutgers University Press, 1988), 59.

36. Moursund, *Medicine in Greater Houston,* 487.

37. Ibid., 489.

38. Ibid., 492–95.

## Chapter 2

1. Thomas D. Anderson, "Anderson Ancestors," unpublished manuscript, September 2003, 4; "1850 Census—Tennessee, Index to the Surname Anderson," transcribed and edited by Byron and Barbara Sistler, n.d., 4; N. Don Macon, *Monroe Dunaway Anderson, His Legacy* (Houston: Texas Medical Center, 1994), 1–2.

2. Macon, *Monroe Dunaway Anderson,* xiii, 2–3.

3. Ibid., 3–4, 15–16.

4. Max H. Jacobs and H. Dick Golding, *Houston and Cotton* (Houston: Max H. Jacobs Agency, 1949), 47.

5. Anderson, "Anderson Ancestors," 14; Macon, *Monroe Dunaway Anderson,* 3–4, 15–16, 18; Thomas Anderson, interview by William H. Kellar, December 11, 2003, and February 9, 2006.

6. Thomas Anderson, interview by William H. Kellar, February 9, 2006.

7. Frank E. Anderson to Monroe Anderson, December 27, 1902; Frank Anderson to Monroe D. Anderson, January 2, 1903; Frank Anderson to Monroe Anderson, April 13, 1903; in Thomas D. Anderson, "Portrait of a Cotton Man," unpublished manuscript, June 15, 2005; Macon, *Monroe Dunaway Anderson,* 18–19.

8. Macon, *Monroe Dunaway Anderson,* 3, 15–16.

9. Frank Anderson to Monroe Anderson, June 29, 1904, in Anderson, "Portrait of a Cotton Man."

10. Gregory A. Fossedal, *Our Finest Hour: Will Clayton, the Marshall Plan, and the*

*Triumph of Democracy* (Stanford, Calif.: Hoover Institution Press, 1993), 15–16; Ellen Clayton Garwood, *Will Clayton: A Short Biography* (Austin: University of Texas Press, 1958), 129; Macon, *Monroe Dunaway Anderson*, 6–7, 10–12.

11. Benjamin Clayton, *Notes on Some Phases of Cotton Operations, 1905–1929* (N.p.: Privately printed by author, 1965), 8–9; Macon, *Monroe Dunaway Anderson*, 13–15.

12. Clayton, *Notes on Some Phases of Cotton Operations*, 3; Macon, *Monroe Dunaway Anderson*, 25–28.

13. Macon, *Monroe Dunaway Anderson*, 27.

14. Garwood, *Will Clayton*, 130–31; Douglas K. Fleming, *Thoughts of a Cotton Man: From Lamar Fleming's Collected Papers* (Seattle: AlphaGraphics, 1994), 2.

15. Clayton, *Notes on Some Phases of Cotton Operations*, 17–19; Macon, *Monroe Dunaway Anderson*, 23–25.

16. Fleming, *Thoughts of a Cotton Man*, 2.

17. Macon, *Monroe Dunaway Anderson*, 25–28.

18. Fleming, *Thoughts of a Cotton Man*, 78–79.

19. Fossedal, *Our Finest Hour*, 27; Garwood, *Will Clayton*, 80–81; Fleming, *Thoughts of a Cotton Man*, 78–79.

20. Fossedal, *Our Finest Hour*, 28–30.

21. Thomas Anderson, interview by William H. Kellar, December 11, 2003; Macon, *Monroe Dunaway Anderson*, 29–32, Fossedal, *Our Finest Hour*, 31; Clayton, *Notes on Some Phases of Cotton Operations*, 20. It is worth noting that Oklahoma was still a territory in 1904 and would not become a state until November 16, 1907.

22. The firm's financial statement dated April 30, 1905, showed assets of $47,950.00 and liabilities of $8,400.00. Anderson, Clayton & Company, "Statement: April 30, 1905," 5, courtesy of W. Merrill Glasgow, now in Special Collections, M. D. Anderson Library, University of Houston.

23. Harris County Historical Society, *Houston: A History & Guide* (Houston: Anson Jones Press, 1942), 259.

24. Frank E. Anderson to Monroe Anderson, August 27, 1906, in Anderson, "Portrait of a Cotton Man"; Thomas Anderson, interview by William H. Kellar, February 9, 2006; Macon, *Monroe Dunaway Anderson*, 32.

25. Macon, *Monroe Dunaway Anderson*, 34–37; T. V. Thompson and Burt Schorr, "The Story of M. D. Anderson," *Houston Press*, June 24, 1958, 7.

26. Macon, *Monroe Dunaway Anderson*, 34–37. Following W. Leland Anderson's death, a cache of forty letters written by his father, Frank E. Anderson, to Monroe D. Anderson was discovered in Leland's desk. Thomas D. Anderson, Leland's brother, assembled a collection of several letters from this cache, with annotations on the others. He wrote: "There were 40 letters from FEA to MDA, several written while MDA was still a banker in Jackson; MDA moved to Houston in 1907 after the credit

demands of the new company outran the lending limits of Jackson's two banks. He may have been unhappy in Houston; FEA's letter of April 22, 1911, expresses surprise that MDA is considering withdrawal from the firm. Of course, it didn't happen." Anderson, "Portrait of a Cotton Man," 9.

27. Ray Miller, *Ray Miller's Houston,* 2nd ed. (Houston: Gulf Publishing, 1992), 52–53; Macon, *Monroe Dunaway Anderson,* 36; Thomas Anderson, interview by William H. Kellar, February 9, 2006.

28. Thomas Anderson, interview by William H. Kellar, February 9, 2006; Macon, *Monroe Dunaway Anderson,* 42; Gail Rickey, "M. D. Anderson: Catalyst behind Major Med Center," *Houston Business Journal,* May 6, 1985; and Thompson and Schorr, "Story of M. D. Anderson," 7.

29. Rickey, "M. D. Anderson"; Thomas Anderson, interview by William H. Kellar, February 9, 2006.

30. Fossedal, *Our Finest Hour,* 23; Thomas Anderson, interview by William H. Kellar, December 11, 2003, and February 9, 2006. While working for American Cotton Company in 1900, Will Clayton had developed appendicitis, and Lamar Fleming brought him to his home to recuperate. Under the Flemings' care, Will not only improved his health but began a new relationship working under Fleming in a newly vacated position. Fleming and Clayton fought against a faction of the American Cotton Company that they believed was taking the company into bankruptcy.

31. Rickey, "M. D. Anderson."

32. Ibid.; Macon, *Monroe Dunaway Anderson,* 56.

33. Thompson and Schorr, "Story of M. D. Anderson," 7; Macon, *Monroe Dunaway Anderson,* 37–38.

34. Thomas Anderson, interview by William H. Kellar, February 9, 2006; Macon, *Monroe Dunaway Anderson,* 49; Miller, *Ray Miller's Houston,* 56–63; Anderson, Clayton & Company, "Financial Statement as of August 4, 1915," "Financial Statement August 12, 1916," Special Collections, M. D. Anderson Library, University of Houston.

35. Fleming, *Thoughts of a Cotton Man,* 79.

36. Anderson, Clayton & Company, "Anderson Clayton: Eight Decades of Progress," *Annual Report 1984,* 4–7; Port of Houston Authority, "Then and Now: Needed Expansion," *Port of Houston Magazine,* May/June 2005, 28–30; Thomas Anderson, interview by William H. Kellar, December 11, 2003; John H. Crooker Jr. and Gibson Gayle Jr., *Fulbright & Jaworski, 75 Years: 1919–1994* (Houston: Fulbright & Jaworski LLP, 1994), 9; Garwood, *Will Clayton,* 95.

37. Anderson, "Portrait of a Cotton Man," 6; Macon, *Monroe Dunaway Anderson,* 52.

38. Thomas D. Anderson, "Official Texas Historical Marker Form—Anderson, Clayton & Co.," 2004, 12, courtesy of Thomas D. Anderson; Anderson, "Portrait of a Cotton Man," 5; Macon, *Monroe Dunaway Anderson,* 51–54.

39. Thomas Anderson, interview by William H. Kellar, December 11, 2003, and February 9, 2006; Macon, *Monroe Dunaway Anderson*, 53–56.

## Chapter 3

1. John H. Crooker Jr. and Gibson Gayle Jr., *Fulbright & Jaworski, 75 Years: 1919–1994* (Houston: Fulbright & Jaworski LLP, 1994), 7; *Texas Almanac 2006–2007* (Dallas: Dallas Morning News, 2006), 180.

2. Crooker and Gayle, *Fulbright & Jaworski*, 8; Newton Gresham and James A. Tinsley, "Fulbright, Rufus Clarence," *Handbook of Texas Online*, http://www.tshaonline.org/handbook/online/articles/ffu19 (accessed January 13, 2011).

3. Crooker and Gayle, *Fulbright & Jaworski*, 8–10.

4. Zarko Franks, "'No Finer Mind, No Finer Heart,' They Say of John Henry Freeman," *Houston Chronicle*, March 3, 1968; John H. Freeman, interview by Don Macon, August 2, 1973; Crooker and Gayle, *Fulbright & Jaworski*, 17.

5. John H. Freeman, interview by Don Macon, August 2, 1973; Crooker and Gayle, *Fulbright & Jaworski*, 17–18; N. Don Macon, *Mr. John H. Freeman and Friends: A Story of the Texas Medical Center and How It Began* (Houston: Texas Medical Center, 1973), 14–16. In 1921, when the State Bank and Trust Company received a national charter, the name was changed to State National Bank. When Freeman joined Fulbright & Crooker in 1924, he brought the bank's account to his new firm, now named Fulbright, Crooker & Freeman.

6. Crooker and Gayle, *Fulbright & Jaworski*, 10–11.

7. Ibid., 11.

8. Ibid., 12.

9. David C. Humphrey, "Prostitution," *Handbook of Texas Online* http://www.tshaonline.org/handbook/online/articles/jbp01 (accessed February 18, 2011); Crooker and Gayle, *Fulbright & Jaworski*, 13; Robert V. Haynes, *A Night of Violence: The Houston Riot of 1917* (Baton Rouge: Louisiana State University Press, 1976), 18–22.

10. Humphrey, "Prostitution"; Haynes, *A Night of Violence*, 18–22.

11. Crooker and Gayle, *Fulbright & Jaworski*, 13; Robert V. Haynes, "Houston Riot of 1917," *Handbook of Texas Online*, http://www.tshaonline.org/handbook/online/articles/jch04 (accessed February 17, 2011). See also Haynes, *A Night of Violence*.

12. Crooker and Gayle, *Fulbright & Jaworski*, 14–15; Bryant Boutwell, "Two Bachelors, a Vision, and the Texas Medical Center, *Houston Review of History and Culture 2*, no. 1 (Fall 2004): 11; Richard Stranahan Ruiz and William Henry Kellar, *Ophthalmology at Hermann Hospital & The University of Texas, Houston: A Personal Perspective* (Houston: Hermann Eye Fund, 2010), 9–11.

13. Crooker and Gayle, *Fulbright & Jaworski*, 15.

14. Harold T. Purvis, "Nat, Texas," *Handbook of Texas Online*, http://www.tsha-online.org/handbook/online/articles/hnn02 (accessed November 19, 2010); N. Don Macon, *South from Flower Mountain: A Conversation with William B. Bates* (Houston: Texas Medical Center, 1975), 18, 20. There is some confusion about whether Bates was born in 1889 or 1890, but Bates told Don Macon in an April 19, 1973, interview that he was born in what became Nat, Texas, in 1889.

15. Macon, *South from Flower Mountain*, 29.

16. Crooker and Gayle, *Fulbright & Jaworski*, 18.

17. William B. Bates, interview by N. Don Macon, April 19, 1973.

18. Ibid.; US Army, *358th Inf., 90th Div., Company E, Sept. 1917, June 1919: American Expeditionary Forces, June 1918, June 1919* (Daun, Germany: A. Schneider, 1919), 2–6.

19. J. Rickard, "Battle of Saint Mihiel, 12–13 September 1918," in *Military History Encyclopedia on the Web*, http://www.historyofwar.org/articles/battles_st_mihiel.html (accessed November 26, 2010); US Army, *358th Inf., 90th Div., Company E*, 6–11.

20. William B. Bates, interview by N. Don Macon, April 19, 1973; US Army, *358th Inf., 90th Div., Company E*, 12–30; Mary Bates Bentsen, interview by William H. Kellar, August 23, 2010.

21. William B. Bates, interview by N. Don Macon, April 19, 1973.

22. Macon, *South from Flower Mountain*, 43–46; Crooker and Gayle, *Fulbright & Jaworski*, 19.

23. Crooker and Gayle, *Fulbright & Jaworski*, 16.

24. William B. Bates, interview by N. Don Macon, April 19, 1973.

25. Ibid.

26. Macon, *South from Flower Mountain*, 52.

27. Ibid., 51–52.

28. William B. Bates, interview by N. Don Macon, April 19, 1973; Macon, *South from Flower Mountain*, 52–53; Crooker and Gayle, *Fulbright & Jaworski*, 16.

29. Macon, *Mr. John H. Freeman and Friends*, 18–19.

30. Macon, *South from Flower Mountain*, 54–55.

31. Ibid., 56–57; William B. Bates, *Monroe D. Anderson: His Life and Legacy*, address delivered at the first annual meeting of the Texas Gulf Coast Historical Association, Houston, November 20, 1956, Publications 1, no. 1 (Houston: Texas Gulf Coast Historical Association, 1957), 5.

## Chapter 4

1. *Estate of Monroe D. Anderson*, 8 T.C. 706 (March 31, 1947), M. D. Anderson Foundation Archives, 707.

2. Benjamin Clayton, *Notes on Some Phases of Cotton Operations, 1905–1929* (N.p.: Privately printed by author, 1965), 1–2; *Estate of Monroe D. Anderson*, 708–709. In 1933 Benjamin Clayton established the Clayton Foundation for Research. See N. Don Macon, *South from Flower Mountain: A Conversation with William B. Bates* (Houston: Texas Medical Center, 1975), 55; C. W. Wellen, president of the Clayton Foundation for Research, interview by William H. Kellar, December 10, 2005.

3. Macon, *South from Flower Mountain*, 57; William B. Bates, interview by N. Don Macon, April 19, 1973; James S. Olson, *Making Cancer History: Disease and Discovery at the University of Texas M. D. Anderson Cancer Center* (Baltimore: Johns Hopkins University Press, 2009), 29.

4. Macon, *South from Flower Mountain*, 72; William B. Bates, interview by N. Don Macon, April 19, 1973.

5. W. B. Bates, "History and Development of the Texas Medical Center," unpublished manuscript, 1956, 3–4, read before the first annual meeting of the Texas Gulf Coast Historical Association, November 20, 1956, John P. McGovern Historical Collections and Research Center, Texas Medical Center Library.

6. "Trust Indenture, Dated July 9, 1936, Creating the M. D. Anderson Foundation," M. D. Anderson Foundation files, 12; William B. Bates, *Monroe D. Anderson: His Life and Legacy*, address delivered at the first annual meeting of the Texas Gulf Coast Historical Association, Houston, November 20, 1956, Publications 1, no. 1 (Houston: Texas Gulf Coast Historical Association, 1957), 5–6.

7. Bates, *Monroe D. Anderson*, 6–7.

8. Thomas D. Anderson, interview by William H. Kellar, December 11, 2003.

9. James Greenwood Jr., *Monroe Dunaway Anderson: Benefactor of Medicine and Mankind* (Austin: Texas Medical Association, 1965), 6; reprinted from *Texas State Journal of Medicine* 61 (May 1965): 414–19.

10. Accounts vary over whether the stroke affected M. D. Anderson's left or right side. The physician who treated him, Dr. James Greenwood Jr., wrote in an article published in 1965 that the stroke affected Anderson's left side. See Greenwood, *Monroe Dunaway Anderson*, 4.

11. N. Don Macon and Thomas Dunaway Anderson, *Monroe Dunaway Anderson, His Legacy: A History of the Texas Medical Center*, 50th Anniversary Edition (Houston: Texas Medical Center, 1994), 65–67; Thomas D. Anderson, interview by William H. Kellar, December 11, 2003; Olson, *Making Cancer History*, 29–30.

12. Macon and Anderson, *Monroe Dunaway Anderson*, 65–67; Thomas D.

Anderson, interview by William H. Kellar, December 11, 2003; Olson, *Making Cancer History*, 29–30.

13. Macon and Anderson, *Monroe Dunaway Anderson*, 67; "M. D. Anderson, Head of Cotton Firm, Dies Here," *Houston Post*, August 7, 1939.

14. Thomas D. Anderson, interview by William H. Kellar, December 11, 2003; Macon and Anderson, *Monroe Dunaway Anderson*, 68; Olson, *Making Cancer History*, 29–30; "President of Famed Cotton Firm Expires," *Houston Chronicle*, August 7, 1939; "M. D. Anderson, Head of Cotton Firm, Dies Here," *Houston Post*, August 7, 1939; "M. D. Anderson Tribute Made," *Houston Post*, August 11, 1939.

15. Thomas D. Anderson, interview by William H. Kellar, December 11, 2003; Macon and Anderson, *Monroe Dunaway Anderson*, 68; "M. D. Anderson, Head of Cotton Firm, Dies Here," *Houston Post*, August 7, 1939; "Houston Loses Outstanding Leaders in Cotton Marketing and Dentistry," *Houston Post*, August 8, 1939; "Anderson's Body Is Forwarded to Jackson, Tenn.," *Houston Chronicle*, August 8, 1939; "Mortuary," *Houston Chronicle*, August 8, 1939.

16. "Anderson Will Leaves Huge Fund to Charity," *Houston Chronicle*, August 11, 1939; "Anderson Will Leaves Fund for Foundation," *Houston Post*, August 11, 1939; "Papers to Create Anderson Trust Charity Filed," *Houston Post*, August 12, 1939; "M. D. Anderson Dedicates Wealth to Permanent Service of Humanity," *Houston Post*, August 13, 1939.

17. Thomas D. Anderson, interview by William H. Kellar, December 11, 2003; Macon and Anderson, *Monroe Dunaway Anderson*, 72, 74.

18. William B. Bates, interview by N. Don Macon, April 19, 1973; N. Don Macon, *South from Flower Mountain*, 58; Macon and Anderson, *Monroe Dunaway Anderson*, 81–82. In 1946 the State National Bank of Houston merged with the First National Bank, where Wilkins served as executive vice president. In addition to serving as a trustee of the M. D. Anderson Foundation, Wilkins was a trustee of the Shriners Hospital for Children, a member of the executive committee of the Texas Medical Center, and had also served as treasurer of the Episcopal Diocese of Texas for many years. Horace Morse Wilkins died at Hermann Hospital on September 13, 1953, at the age of sixty-eight. See *Houston Chronicle*, September 14, 1953; *Houston Post*, September 15, 1953.

19. Bates, *Monroe D. Anderson*, 7; William B. Bates, interview by N. Don Macon, April 19, 1973.

20. In 1960 the Sloan-Kettering Institute and Memorial Hospital united to form the Memorial Sloan-Kettering Cancer Center. Today the M. D. Anderson Cancer Center and Memorial Sloan-Kettering Cancer Center are consistently rated as the no. 1 and no. 2 cancer hospitals in the United States. Memorial Sloan-Kettering Cancer Center, "History & Overview," http://www.mskcc.org/mskcc/html/511.cfm (accessed August 1, 2011); *US News and World Report*, "Top-Ranked Hospitals for

Cancer," http://health.usnews.com/best-hospitals/rankings/cancer (accessed December 7, 2011).

21. Olson, *Making Cancer History*, 31; Frederick C. Elliott, interview by William D. Seybold, August 9, 1971; N. Don Macon, *Mr. John H. Freeman and Friends: A Story of the Texas Medical Center and How It Began* (Houston: Texas Medical Center, 1973), 25–27.

22. R. W. Cumley and Joan McCay, eds., *The First Twenty Years of the University of Texas M. D. Anderson Hospital and Tumor Institute* (Houston: University of Texas M. D. Anderson Hospital and Tumor Institute, 1964), 5–17; Macon, *Mr. John H. Freeman and Friends*, 26.

23. Cumley and McCay, eds. *First Twenty Years*, 5–17; Olson, *Making Cancer History*, 32–33.

24. Frederick C. Elliott, *The Birth of the Texas Medical Center: A Personal Account*, edited by William Henry Kellar (College Station: Texas A&M University Press, 2004), 61–68.

25. Macon, *Mr. John H. Freeman and Friends*, 23–25.

26. William B. Bates, interview by N. Don Macon, April 19, 1973; Macon, *Mr. John H. Freeman and Friends*, 26–27.

27. William B. Bates, interview by N. Don Macon, April 19, 1973; Bates, *Monroe D. Anderson*, 7–8; Macon, *South from Flower Mountain*, 59–61; Kate Sayen Kirkland, *The Hogg Family and Houston: Philanthropy and the Civic Ideal* (Austin: University of Texas Press, 2009), 60; Elliott, *Birth of the Texas Medical Center*, 69–70.

28. Macon and Anderson, *Monroe Dunaway Anderson*, 88–90.

29. Bates, *Monroe D. Anderson*, 5.

## Chapter 5

1. N. Don Macon and Thomas Dunaway Anderson, *Monroe Dunaway Anderson, His Legacy: A History of the Texas Medical Center*, 50th Anniversary Edition (Houston: Texas Medical Center, 1994), 88–90; James S. Olson, *Making Cancer History: Disease and Discovery at the University of Texas M. D. Anderson Cancer Center* (Baltimore: Johns Hopkins University Press, 2009), 33.

2. Spies was accused of having the school's main switchboard tapped and of being "immoral, dictatorial, professionally incompetent, verbally abusive, responsible for the suicides of two faculty members, a sex pervert, a thief, an anti-Semitic Fascist, a communist, a Nazi sympathizer, a homosexual," and of having been forced to leave his previous position in India because of "his lecherous behavior with the wives of his professional associates." Controversy continued on the University of Texas campus, and within four years, the same fate would befall UT president Homer Rainey. Dr. Chauncey D. Leake replaced John Spies in charge of the medical school, and in 1946

Dr. Theophilus S. Painter took over after Rainey's dismissal. See Don E. Carleton, *A Breed So Rare: The Life of J. R. Parten, Liberal Texas Oil Man, 1896–1992* (Austin: Texas State Historical Association, 1998), 226–33; *The University of Texas Medical Branch at Galveston: A Seventy-five Year History by the Faculty and Staff* (Austin: University of Texas Press, 1967) 163–68; Chester Burns, interview by William H. Kellar, July 16, 2001.

3. Frederick C. Elliott, *The Birth of the Texas Medical Center: A Personal Account*, edited by William Henry Kellar (College Station: Texas A&M University Press, 2004), 75–76, 84–85.

4. William D. Seybold, transcript of telephone conversation with Robert A. Shepherd, June 17, 1971, 1, William D. Seybold Papers, John P. McGovern Historical Collections and Research Center, Texas Medical Center Library; Heather Green Wooten, notes for unpublished biography of E. W. Bertner, 9.

5. Janet Schmelzer, "Campbell, Thomas Mitchell," *Handbook of Texas Online*, http://www.tshaonline.org/handbook/online/articles/fca37 (accessed August 27, 2011). The Robertson law was finally repealed in May 1963.

6. William D. Seybold, *E. W. Bertner, M.D., F.A.C.S.: Cancer Fighter* (presidential address to the Texas Surgical Society, Waco, Texas, October 4, 1971), photocopy in William D. Seybold Papers, John P. McGovern Historical Collections and Research Center, Texas Medical Center Library; Gus Bertner to William Spencer Carter (or State Medical Institute), November 20, 1907; William Spencer Carter to Gus Bertner, November 23, 1907, Dean's Office Records, series 1, box 1, Correspondence: 1904–1908, folder: 1907, A–C, Blocker History of Medicine Collections, Moody Medical Library.

7. University of Texas Medical Branch, Dean's Office Records, Sessions 1908–1909, 1909–1910, and 1910–1911, Blocker History of Medicine Collections, Moody Medical Library; Chester R. Burns, *Saving Lives, Training Caregivers, Making Discoveries: A Centennial History of the University of Texas Medical Branch at Galveston* (Austin: Texas State Historical Association, 2003), 182; *University of Texas Medical Branch at Galveston*, 30.

8. William D. Seybold, interview by William H. Kellar, November 14, 2000; Seybold, *E. W. Bertner*, 2; Heather Wooten, "Johnson Interview with E. W. Bertner," notes for unpublished biography of E. W. Bertner, 5–7. Jesse Jones's new Rice Hotel opened on May 17, 1913.

9. Seybold, *E. W. Bertner*, 4–5.

10. Ibid., 6; Olson, *Making Cancer History*, 28; Army of the United States of America, Certificate of Honorable Discharge, April 19, 1919, Form No. 525-2. A. G. O., courtesy of Julie Thurmond.

11. "Houstonians Sail for Visit in the Old World," *Houston Chronicle*, June 1, 1937; Seybold, *E. W. Bertner*.

12. N. Don Macon, *Mr. John H. Freeman and Friends: A Story of the Texas Medical Center and How It Began* (Houston: Texas Medical Center, 1973), 36.

13. Ibid., 27–28; William B. Bates, interview by N. Don Macon, April 19, 1973.

14. William B. Bates, interview by N. Don Macon, April 19, 1973; William B. Bates, *Monroe D. Anderson: His Life and Legacy*, address delivered at the first annual meeting of the Texas Gulf Coast Historical Association, Houston, November 20, 1956, Publications 1, no. 1 (Houston: Texas Gulf Coast Historical Association, 1957), 9. Bates stated that after the war, "to add to these facilities, Mr. and Mrs. Lamar Fleming Jr., acquired and donated a two-story apartment dwelling at 406 Webster Street, which, when converted to convalescent quarters, greatly augmented the size of accommodations at the disposition of the clinic" (Bates, *Monroe D. Anderson*, 9). See R. W. Cumley and Joan McCay, eds., *The First Twenty Years of the University of Texas M. D. Anderson Hospital and Tumor Institute* (Houston: University of Texas M. D. Anderson Hospital and Tumor Institute, 1964), 50–51.

15. Olson, *Making Cancer History*, 33–34; Cumley and McCay, eds., *First Twenty Years*, 28–51; Elliott, *Birth of the Texas Medical Center*, 76.

16. Bates, *Monroe D. Anderson*, 11–12; N. Don Macon, *South from Flower Mountain: A Conversation with William B. Bates* (Houston: Texas Medical Center, 1975), 64–65; E. W. D'Anton, *Memories: A History of the University of Texas Dental Branch at Houston* (Houston: University of Texas Health Science Center at Houston Dental Branch, 1991), 21–22; Elliott, *Birth of the Texas Medical Center*, 76–78.

17. Macon, *Mr. John H. Freeman and Friends*, 27–28; William B. Bates, interview by N. Don Macon, April 19, 1973; Elliott, *Birth of the Texas Medical Center*, 76–78, 83. As Elliott wrote: "September 1, 1943, was a new day at the dental school. It was the close of the Texas Dental College and the opening of the University of Texas Dental Branch."

## Chapter 6

1. Years later, in November 1950, Carr P. Collins recorded his recollections of what happened next in a letter to Earl C. Hankamer. In 1959 D. K. Martin provided his account in a letter to Guy B. Harrison, a history professor at Baylor University. These two letters provide valuable insight from two of the key figures in the events that ultimately led to moving Baylor College of Medicine to Houston. Walter H. Moursund, dean of the Baylor College of Medicine at the time, recalled events from his perspective after he retired. See *A History of Baylor University College of Medicine, 1900–1953* (Houston: Gulf Printing, 1956).

2. Baylor College of Medicine, "BCM History," http://www.bcm.edu/about/history.cfm (accessed September 9, 2011); Ruth SoRelle, *The Quest for Excellence: Baylor College of Medicine, 1900–2000* (Houston: Baylor College of Medicine, 2000), 37–39.

3. SoRelle, *Quest for Excellence*, 41–42; William T. Butler, interview by William H. Kellar, September 9, 2010; Randy J. Sparks, "Moursund, Walter Henrik," *Handbook*

*of Texas Online*, http://www.tshaonline.org/handbook/online/articles/fm087 (accessed October 10, 2011).

4. Moursund, *History of Baylor University College of Medicine*, 102.

5. Ibid., 108–10.

6. D. K. Martin to Guy B. Harrison, Baylor University, Waco, Texas, February 18, 1959, M. D. Anderson Foundation files.

7. Ibid.

8. N. Don Macon, *Mr. John H. Freeman and Friends: A Story of the Texas Medical Center and How It Began* (Houston: Texas Medical Center, 1973), 44.

9. Carr P. Collins to Earl C. Hankamer, November 16, 1950, M. D. Anderson Foundation Archives.

10. N. Don Macon, *South from Flower Mountain: A Conversation with William B. Bates* (Houston: Texas Medical Center, 1975), 63.

11. Collins to Hankamer, November 16, 1950.

12. Ibid.; Martin to Harrison, February 18, 1959; Macon, *Mr. John H. Freeman and Friends*, 44.

13. "Baylor Cancels Contract to Join Medical Foundation: Is Acceptable to Center; Church Insists on Control; Houston Invites College," *Dallas Morning News*, April 28, 1943; Carr P. Collins, "Withdrawal from Foundation and Removal of Baylor to Houston Explained by Trustee," *Dallas Morning News*, May 15, 1943; SoRelle, *Quest for Excellence*, 43; Moursund, *History of Baylor University College of Medicine*, 111–12.

14. M. D. Anderson Foundation to Board of Trustees, Baylor University, May 5, 1943, Baylor College of Medicine Archives, M. D. Anderson Foundation File, courtesy of William T. Butler, MD.

15. Moursund, *History of Baylor University College of Medicine*, 114–17. Moursund wrote: "In 1943, the Southwestern Medical Foundation established a medical college, the Southwestern Medical College, in a temporary building near Parkland Hospital in Dallas. Effective September 1, 1949, the Southwestern Medical Foundation ceased operating the Southwestern Medical College and transferred all of its facilities to the University of Texas."

16. William B. Bates, *Monroe D. Anderson: His Life and Legacy*, address delivered at the first annual meeting of the Texas Gulf Coast Historical Association, Houston, November 20, 1956, Publications 1, no. 1 (Houston: Texas Gulf Coast Historical Association, 1957), 11; Macon, *South from Flower Mountain*, 64; Moursund, *History of Baylor University College of Medicine*, 117–18.

17. William T. Butler, interview by William H. Kellar, September 9, 2010. Dr. Butler is chancellor emeritus and former president of Baylor College of Medicine.

18. Frederick C. Elliott, *The Birth of the Texas Medical Center: A Personal Account*, edited by William Henry Kellar (College Station: Texas A&M University Press, 2004), 81; Macon, *Mr. John H. Freeman and Friends*, 48.

19. Moursund, *History of Baylor University College of Medicine*, 118.

20. Harris County Medical Society, "Minutes of the Meeting of the Fact Finding Committee held May 14, 1943," John P. McGovern Historical Collections and Research Center, Texas Medical Center Library.

21. Ibid.

22. Ibid.; Harris County Medical Society, *A History of Organized Medicine in Harris County, Texas* (Houston, 1948), 14–15; "Harris County Medical Society Welcomes Baylor to Houston," *Houston Post*, July 31, 1943.

23. Earl C. Hankamer, interview by N. Don Macon, October 9, 1973. N. Don Macon and Thomas Dunaway Anderson, *Monroe Dunaway Anderson, His Legacy: A History of the Texas Medical Center*, 50th Anniversary Edition (Houston: Texas Medical Center, 1994), 94–96; Macon, *Mr. John H. Freeman and Friends*, 45–47; "Group Named on Moving of College Here," unidentified clipping, May 1943, M. D. Anderson Foundation files; Baylor College of Medicine, "BCM History," http://www.bcm.edu/about/history.cfm (accessed September 9, 2011).

24. "School's Move to Houston Well Advised," *Houston Post*, July 31, 1943.

25. Macon and Anderson, *Monroe Dunaway Anderson*, 88–90.

26. "22 to 1 Majority Favors Sale of Tract Near Park," *Houston Post*, December 15, 1943; "Voters Approve Land Sale; Only 951 Ballots Cast," *Houston Chronicle*, December 15, 1943; Macon, *South from Flower Mountain*, 62; Bates, *Monroe D. Anderson*, 10; *Houston Post*, April 20, 1944; Macon and Anderson, *Monroe Dunaway Anderson*, 140.

27. William T. Butler, interview by William H. Kellar, September 9, 2010; W. B. Bates, "History and Development of the Texas Medical Center," unpublished manuscript, 1956, 10, read before the first annual meeting of the Texas Gulf Coast Historical Association, November 20, 1956, John P. McGovern Historical Collections and Research Center, Texas Medical Center Library.

## Chapter 7

1. Julia Bertner Naylor, interview by N. Don Macon, July 19, 1973; Anna Hanselman, interview by Dr. William D. Seybold, May 16, 1970.

2. "M. D. Anderson Cancer Hospital Dedicated," *Houston Magazine* 16, no. 2 (March 1944): 4–8; Helen T. Konjias, ed. *The Manual of the M. D. Anderson Hospital for Cancer Research* (Houston: M. D. Anderson Hospital Publications, University of Texas, 1945), 188.

3. Anna Hanselman, interview by Dr. William D. Seybold, May 16, 1970.

4. Julia Bertner Naylor, interview by N. Don Macon, July 19, 1973; Anna Hanselman, interview by Dr. William D. Seybold, May 16, 1970; Marguerite Johnston, *Houston: The Unknown City, 1836–1946* (College Station: Texas A&M University Press, 1991), 193–94, 230; "Plans for Southwest's Greatest Medical Center

Progress," *Houston Magazine*, 16 (August 1944); Frederick C. Elliott, *The Birth of the Texas Medical Center: A Personal Account*, edited by William Henry Kellar (College Station: Texas A&M University Press, 2004), 80.

5. Elliott, *The Birth of the Texas Medical Center*, 84–85; H. H. Weinert, Orville Bullington, and D. F. Strickland, "Medical Committee Report to the Board of Regents of the University of Texas," September 29, 1944, M. D. Anderson Foundation files.

6. "Plans for Southwest's Greatest Medical Center Progress."

7. Elliott, *Birth of the Texas Medical Center*, 85; Weinert, Bullington, and Strickland, "Medical Committee Report to the Board of Regents," 11–12.

8. George Norris Green, *The Establishment in Texas Politics: The Primitive Years, 1938–1957* (Norman: University of Oklahoma Press, 1979), 83, 86–87; Don E. Carleton, *A Breed So Rare: The Life of J. R. Parten, Liberal Texas Oil Man, 1896–1992* (Austin: Texas State Historical Association, 1998), 300–306.

9. Elliott, *Birth of the Texas Medical Center*, 87–88; Frederick C. Elliott, interview by William D. Seybold, August 9, 1971; "Bertner Tours Med Ctr," *Houston Post*, December 6, 1944, 8; "Med Ctr Discussed by Director," *Houston Chronicle*, December 5, 1944, 11. The story has become part of the legend and lore of the Texas Medical Center, and yet there is some confusion about whether Bertner made his famous speech in December of 1944 or 1945 and to whom he spoke. Frederick Elliott recalled the story of Bertner's speech years later. He said that Bertner had called him in November, saying that he had been invited to speak at the Kiwanis Club at their first meeting in December. But evidence suggests that it was not the Kiwanis Club but the Southampton Civic Club, which held its monthly meeting on December 4, 1944, at Edgar Allen Poe Elementary School, that provided Bertner's audience. Elliott also told William D. Seybold that the event took place in December 1945, but there are no published accounts of Bertner giving this speech at that time. According to Elliott, the next morning the *Houston Post* printed a full-page headline, "$100 Million Medical Center for Houston." But the only evidence is an article that appeared in the *Houston Chronicle*, "Medic Center Is Discussed by Director." What is known is that an article in one of the Houston newspapers caught the eye of William B. Bates, and his ensuing conversation with Elliott has been related by others. It is possible that Elliott confused the date and occasion in his reminiscences when he wrote his memoir. By the end of 1944, it was common for Bertner to talk about the future "$100 million" Texas Medical Center.

10. "Dr. Bertner Is Medical Center Chief," *Houston Chronicle*, December 12, 1945; William B. Bates, *Monroe D. Anderson: His Life and Legacy*, address delivered at the first annual meeting of the Texas Gulf Coast Historical Association, Houston, November 20, 1956, Publications 1, no. 1 (Houston: Texas Gulf Coast Historical Association, 1957), 8–9; N. Don Macon, *South from Flower Mountain: A Conversation with William B. Bates* (Houston: Texas Medical Center, 1975), 67–69; Elliott, *Birth of the Texas Medical Center*, 86.

11. Jim Carroll, "Great Future for Medical Center Painted at Dedicatory

Banquet," *Houston Press*, March 1, 1946; N. Don Macon, *Mr. John H. Freeman and Friends: A Story of the Texas Medical Center and How It Began* (Houston: Texas Medical Center, 1973), 49–50; "Dedicatory Proceedings of the Texas Medical Center, February 28, 1946," courtesy of Mavis P. Kelsey, MD.

12. Carroll, "Great Future for Medical Center Painted at Dedicatory Banquet," March 1, 1946.

13. "New Gift to Big Medical Center Made," *Houston Chronicle*, March 3, 1946; Macon, *South from Flower Mountain*, 66–67.

14. Macon, *South from Flower Mountain*, 62, 67–69; Macon, *Mr. John H. Freeman and Friends*, 47–48; Bates, *Monroe D. Anderson*, 10.

15. N. Don Macon, *Clark and the Anderson: A Personal Profile*, (Houston: Texas Medical Center, 1976), 138–42.

16. Ibid., 146–56, 158–61; Ochsner Health System, "Ochsner Timeline: 1940s," http://academics.ochsner.org/librarypro.aspx?id=17018 (accessed March 7, 2012). See also Alton Ochsner, "Primary Pulmonary Malignancy," *Surgery, Gynecology and Obstetrics* 68 (1939): 435–51.

17. R. W. Cumley and Joan McCay, eds., *The First Twenty Years of the University of Texas M. D. Anderson Hospital and Tumor Institute* (Houston: University of Texas M. D. Anderson Hospital and Tumor Institute, 1964), 50–55.

18. William D. Seybold, *E. W. Bertner, M.D., F.A.C.S.: Cancer Fighter* (presidential address to the Texas Surgical Society, Waco, Texas, October 4, 1971), 9, photocopy in William D. Seybold Papers, John P. McGovern Historical Collections and Research Center, Texas Medical Center Library.

19. Texas Medical Center, "TMC History 1945–1954," http://www.texasmedicalcenter.org/root/en/GetToKnow/History/1945–1954.htm (accessed January 20, 2012); "Plans for Southwest's Greatest Medical Center Progress."

20. Later in 1948 Dr. Michael E. DeBakey joined the faculty as chair of the department of surgery. See William T. Butler, interview by William H. Kellar, September 9, 2010; Baylor College of Medicine, "BCM History," http://www.bcm.edu/about/history.cfm (accessed September 9, 2011); Texas Medical Center, "TMC History 1945–1954."

21. Texas Medical Center, "TMC History 1945–1954."

22. Dudley Y. Oldham, interview notes by William D. Seybold, July 9, 1971; National Center for Biotechnology Information, US National Library of Medicine, "A.D.A.M. Medical Encyclopedia: Rhabdomyosarcoma," http://www.ncbi.nlm.nih.gov/pubmedhealth/PMH0002402/ (accessed February 17, 2012).

23. Dudley Y. Oldham, interview notes by William D. Seybold, July 9, 1971.

24. Mavis P. Kelsey, *Twentieth-Century Doctor: House Calls to Space Medicine* (College Station: Texas A&M University Press, 1999), 201–202; Seybold, *E. W. Bertner*; William D. Seybold, interview by William H. Kellar, November 14, 2000; Dudley Y. Oldham, interview notes by William D. Seybold, July 9, 1971.

25. James S. Olson, *Making Cancer History: Disease and Discovery at the University of Texas M. D. Anderson Cancer Center* (Baltimore: Johns Hopkins University Press, 2009), 39–40; Kelsey, *Twentieth-Century Doctor,* 201–202; Seybold, *E. W. Bertner;* William D. Seybold, interview by William H. Kellar, November 14, 2000; Dudley Y. Oldham, interview notes by William D. Seybold, July 9, 1971.

26. Olson, *Making Cancer History,* 39–40, 57.

27. Cornelius P. Rhoads to E. W. Bertner, received by TMC on May 22, 1950, Ernst W. Bertner Papers, Manuscript Collection 2, John P. McGovern Historical Collections and Research Center, Texas Medical Center Library.

28. John H. Freeman, interview notes by William D. Seybold, April 8, 1971.

29. Seybold, *E. W. Bertner,* 11.

30. Dudley Y. Oldham, interview notes by William D. Seybold, July 9, 1971.

## Chapter 8

1. N. Don Macon, *South from Flower Mountain: A Conversation with William B. Bates* (Houston: Texas Medical Center, 1975), 67–69; Frederick C. Elliott, *The Birth of the Texas Medical Center: A Personal Account,* edited by William Henry Kellar (College Station: Texas A&M University Press, 2004), 133.

2. R. W. Cumley and Joan McCay, eds., *The First Twenty Years of the University of Texas M. D. Anderson Hospital and Tumor Institute* (Houston: University of Texas M. D. Anderson Hospital and Tumor Institute, 1964), 67–69; James S. Olson, *Making Cancer History: Disease and Discovery at the University of Texas M. D. Anderson Cancer Center* (Baltimore: Johns Hopkins University Press, 2009), 56–57.

3. *Houston Chronicle,* January 26, 1951; *Houston Chronicle,* May 23, 1951; Betsy Parish, *Legacy—50 Years of Loving Care: Texas Children's Hospital, 1954–2004* (Houston: Elisha Freeman Publishing, 2008), 20; E. W. D'Anton, *Memories: A History of the University of Texas Dental Branch at Houston* (Houston: University of Texas Health Science Center at Houston, 1991), 26.

4. Marilyn McAdams Sibley, *The Methodist Hospital of Houston: Serving the World* (Austin: Texas State Historical Association, 1989), 119–20, 133; Elliott, *Birth of the Texas Medical Center,* 128–29.

5. *Houston Chronicle,* October 16, 1952; *Houston Post,* October 16, 1952; *Houston Press,* October 16, 1952; Kimberly Youngblood, "The Houston Academy of Medicine—Texas Medical Center Library: A Notable Medical Athenaeum," *Houston Review of History and Culture* 2, no. 1 (Fall 2004): 31–32.

6. Rosanne Clark, "Texas Medical Center Celebrates 50 Years of Visions Fulfilled: The Early Fifties Bring Continued Growth," *Texas Medical Center News,* February 15, 1995, 11; "Huge Texas Medical Center Makes Progress in Houston," *American City,* February 1952, 114–15; Elliott, *Birth of the Texas Medical Center,* 130–31; D'Anton, *Memories,* 26–27.

7. Elliott, *Birth of the Texas Medical Center*, 133–34.

8. *Houston Chronicle*, October 1, 1952; *Houston Post*, October 1, 1952; *Houston Press*, October 1, 1952; Elliott, *Birth of the Texas Medical Center*, 133–34.

9. Frederick Chesley Elliott: Biographical Data, Elliott Papers, John P. McGovern Historical Collections and Research Center, Texas Medical Center Library.

10. Frederick C. Elliott, interview by William D. Seybold, August 9, 1971. History Committee, Delta Sigma Delta, *History of Delta Sigma Delta Fraternity, 1882–1946* (N.p.: 1950), 246.

11. Cumley and McCay, eds., *First Twenty Years*, 69, 84; Elliott, *Birth of the Texas Medical Center*, 135.

12. "H. M. Wilkins, Veteran Banker and Civic Leader Here, Dies," *Houston Chronicle*, September 14, 1953; W. B. Bates, "History and Development of the Texas Medical Center," unpublished manuscript, 1956, 5, read before the first annual meeting of the Texas Gulf Coast Historical Association, November 20, 1956, John P. McGovern Historical Collections and Research Center, Texas Medical Center Library.

13. E. L. Summers, "Anderson Foundation Putting Out 14 Millions, Finds Assets Soaring, *Houston Chronicle*, February 14, 1954; Bates, "History and Development of the Texas Medical Center," 6.

14. Cumley and McCay, eds., *First Twenty Years*, 74–89; Elliott, *The Birth of the Texas Medical Center: A Personal Account*, 148; Olson, *Making Cancer History*, 61–62.

15. Cumley and McCay, eds., *First Twenty Years*, 89–94; Elliott, *Birth of the Texas Medical Center*, 148; Olson, *Making Cancer History*, 61–62.

16. *Houston Chronicle*, September 10, 1954; *Houston Post*, September 10, 1954; Youngblood, "Houston Academy of Medicine," 32.

17. Elliott, *Birth of the Texas Medical Center*, 147–48; "The Plan of Campaign for the Parish: St. Luke's Episcopal Hospital, Diocese of Texas" (approved by the 98th Council at Beaumont, Texas, January 27, 1946), M. D. Anderson Foundation files. On January 27, 1946, the 98th Council of the Episcopal Diocese of Texas approved a $1 million, statewide fund-raising plan for St. Luke's Episcopal Hospital, to be built in the new Texas Medical Center in Houston. The previous October, the 97th Council of the Diocese of Texas adopted St. Luke's Episcopal Hospital as a Diocesan institution, and the Clergy Conference formally welcomed and endorsed the plans for the new hospital, pledging their enthusiastic support for the plans.

18. D'Anton, *Memories*, 31–33; Elliott, *Birth of the Texas Medical Center*, 151; *Houston Chronicle*, November 27, December 1 and 4, 1955; *Houston Post*, November 30, December 1 and 2, 1955.

19. On February 26, 1960, Houston Endowment, Inc., made a grant of $100,000 to the Institute of Religion to help finish funding for its building, which at the time was under construction. *Houston Chronicle*, February 27, 1960; *Houston Post*, February 27, 1960.

20. Elliott, *Birth of the Texas Medical Center*, 154; Cumley and McCay, eds., *First*

*Twenty Years,* 95–96, 120. The University of Texas board of regents created the University Cancer Foundation in October 1955 as a nonprofit foundation for "educational and scientific purposes."

21. Bates, "History and Development of the Texas Medical Center," 12–15.

22. TIRR later became the Institute for Rehabilitation and Research. Today it is part of the Memorial Hermann Healthcare System and is known as TIRR-Memorial Hermann.

23. *Houston Post,* July 24, 1958. See also *Houston Press,* July 18, 1958; Elliott, *Birth of the Texas Medical Center,* 166; Texas Trauma Institute, Memorial Hermann, "Life Fight," http://www.memorialhermann.org/specialtyservices/emergencyservices/content.aspx?id=1774 (accessed January 31, 2012).

24. Leon Jaworski had a distinguished career and served as a trustee of the M. D. Anderson Foundation and the Texas Medical Center. He also was president of the State Bar of Texas, American Bar Association, and American College of Trial Lawyers; on November 1, 1973, he was appointed as special prosecutor during the Watergate investigations of the Nixon presidency. In 1974 the firm changed its name to Fulbright & Jaworski, the name by which it is known today. Leon Jaworski died on December 9, 1982, while chopping wood at his ranch near Wimberley, Texas. See John H. Crooker Jr. and Gibson Gayle Jr., *Fulbright & Jaworski, 75 Years: 1919–1994* (Houston: Fulbright & Jaworski LLP, 1994), 139.

25. Ruth SoRelle, *The Quest for Excellence: Baylor College of Medicine, 1900–2000* (Houston: Baylor College of Medicine, 2000), 101–102, 105; Elliott, *Birth of the Texas Medical Center,* 170–72; *Houston Post,* March 13, 1959. In addition to being a Baylor alumnus, Leon Jaworski had other ties to Baylor University through his brother, Dr. Hannibal Jaworski, a surgeon, who graduated from Baylor University College of Medicine in 1924, when it was located in Dallas.

26. Elliott, *Birth of the Texas Medical Center,* 180–81; *Houston Chronicle,* February 18, 19, 1960.

27. *Houston Chronicle,* May 22, 1960; Elliott, *Birth of the Texas Medical Center,* 183–85.

28. Elliott, *Birth of the Texas Medical Center,* 184–86; *Houston Chronicle,* June 2, 1960; Sibley, *Methodist Hospital of Houston,* 149; *Houston Press,* June 3, 1960; *Houston Chronicle,* June 6, 1960; *Houston Chronicle,* August 25, 1960. On racial integration at the UT Dental Branch, see Elliott, *Birth of the Texas Medical Center,* 133 and 217n7. See also William Henry Kellar, *Make Haste Slowly: Moderates, Conservatives, and School Desegregation in Houston* (College Station: Texas A&M University Press, 1999), 119–37.

29. Elliott, *Birth of the Texas Medical Center,* 188. Voters finally approved the Harris County Hospital District in a referendum in November 1965. On January 1, 1966, the Harris County Hospital District was officially established, taking possession and

responsibility for the two city-county hospitals, Jefferson Davis and Ben Taub. The new hospital district was classified as a political subdivision with the authority to levy taxes. Harris Health System, "A Proud History of Caring," https://www.hchdonline.com/en/about-us/who-we-are/pages/history.aspx (accessed January 30, 2012).

30. Elliott, *Birth of the Texas Medical Center*, 188, 192, 194.

31. John H. Freeman, interview notes by William D. Seybold, April 8, 1971.

## Chapter 9

1. Texas Medical Center, *Facts & Figures* (Houston: Texas Medical Center, 2012).

2. Thermal Energy Corporation, *Energy Innovation: A Bridge to the Future—2011 Annual Report* (Houston: TECO, 2012), 12; Texas Medical Center, *Facts & Figures*; Texas Medical Center, "The Texas Medical Center," http://www.texasmedicalcenter.org/about-tmc/ (accessed July 28, 2013).

3. Richard E. Wainerdi, interview by William H. Kellar, May 10, 2012; Bill Mintz and Ruth SoRelle, "St. Luke's Deal Draws Court Action/Med Center Objects to For-profit Alliance," *Houston Chronicle*, May 11, 1996.

4. Jennifer Darwin, "OrNda Signs Memorial Deal, Eyes Affiliation with Hermann: Hospital Firm Seeks Bigger Share of Local Market," *Houston Business Journal*, July 21, 1996, http://www.bizjournals.com/houston/stories/1996/07/22/story3.html?page=all (accessed May 14, 2012).

5. One of the questions about the lawsuit centered on whether the charter and covenants expired after fifty years from the time when the medical center was first established. The Texas Non-Profit Corporation Act (Article 1396-1.01 et seq., Vernon's Texas Civil Statutes), enacted in 1959, made them perpetual for every nonprofit organization in Texas:

Art. 1396–2.02. General Powers

A. Subject to the provisions of Sections B and C of this Article, each corporation shall have power:

(1) To have perpetual succession by its corporate name, unless a limited period of duration is stated in its articles of incorporation. Notwithstanding the articles of incorporation, the period of duration for any corporation incorporated before August 10, 1959, is perpetual if all fees and franchise taxes have been paid as provided by law.

6. Jennifer Darwin, "Settled Suit Leaves Columbia in Limbo: Chain Ponders Inner-City Hospital as Court Stymies St. Luke's Deal," *Houston Business Journal*, August 25, 1996, http://www.bizjournals.com/houston/stories/1996/08/26/story3.html?page=all (accessed May 14, 2012).

7. Bill Mintz, "Big Merger of Houston Hospitals: Memorial Healthcare to Join with Hermann," *Houston Chronicle*, July 1, 1997; "Memorial, Hermann Complete

Merger," *Houston Chronicle*, November 5, 1997. Information on OrNda and Tenet is from "Company Overview of Tenet HealthSystem HealthCorp., Inc.," *Bloomberg Businessweek*, http://investing.businessweek.com/research/stocks/private/snapshot. asp?privcapId=32534 (accessed June 1, 2012).

8. "TMC Purchases Nabisco Facility," *Houston Business Journal*, April 30, 2000, http://www.bizjournals.com/houston/stories/2000/05/01/focus5.html (accessed June 3, 2012).

9. In 1961 Hurricane Carla ravaged the region. Fifteen years later, heavy rains on June 15, 1976, damaged several buildings in the Texas Medical Center and surrounding parts of Harris County. On August 18, 1983, Hurricane Alicia made landfall during the early-morning hours and dropped about five inches of rain over most of the city, but the major damage came from the wind, which gusted to 127 mph. In all, Hurricane Alicia resulted in the deaths of twenty-one persons, destroyed 2,300 homes, and caused about $2 billion in damages across Texas. "Hurricane Alicia, 1983," *USA Today*, September 21, 2005, http://www.usatoday.com/weather/hurricane/history/walicia.htm (accessed June 6, 2012); Committee on Natural Disasters, Commission on Engineering and Technical Systems, National Research Council, *Hurricane Alicia: Galveston and Houston, Texas, August 17–18, 1983,* (Washington, DC: National Academy Press, 1984).

10. Harris County Flood Control District, "Tropical Storm Allison Overview," http://www.hcfcd.org/F_tsa_overview.html (accessed June 4, 2012); Texas Medical Center, "The Texas Medical Center."

11. Clifford Krauss and James C. Mckinley Jr., "Texas Assesses Damage after Hurricane Ike," *New York Times*, September 14, 2008; Richard E. Wainerdi, "From the President," *Texas Medical Center News*, October 15, 2008.

12. National Aeronautics and Space Administration Authorization Act of 2010, Pub. L. No. 111-267, § 1208, 124 Stat. 2845 (2010); Texas Medical Center, *The National Center for Human Performance* (Houston: Texas Medical Center, 2010).

13. Ruth SoRelle, *The Quest for Excellence: Baylor College of Medicine, 1900–2000* (Houston: Baylor College of Medicine, 2000), 110.

14. Ibid., 145; Baylor College of Medicine, "Fast Facts & Figures," http://www. bcm.edu/about/fastfacts.cfm (accessed June 6, 2012); Menninger Clinic, "Houston Becomes Epicenter for Mental Health Research and Treatment . . . ," http://www. menningerclinic.com/about/newsroom/recent-news/menninger-relocates-to-50-acre-hospital-near-texas-medical-center (accessed May 28, 2012).

15. Bryant Boutwell and John P. McGovern, *Conversation with a Medical School: The University of Texas–Houston Medical School, 1970–2000* (Houston: University of Texas–Houston Health Science Center, 1999), 13–15. The health science center also includes the University of Texas Harris County Psychiatric Center, the Mental Sciences Institute, the Brown Foundation Institute of Molecular Medicine for the Prevention of Human Diseases, and several interdisciplinary centers.

16. University of Texas Medical School at Houston, "About Us," http://med.uth.tmc.edu/about-us.htm (accessed May 23, 2012).

17. Texas Woman's University, "About the Houston Center," http://www.twu.edu/houston/about-houston-center.asp (accessed May 16, 2012).

18. Prairie View A&M University, "About the College," http://www.pvamu.edu/pages/1007.asp (accessed May 23, 2012).

19. Texas Medical Center, "The Texas Medical Center"; University of Houston, "Biomedical Engineering," http://www.bioe.uh.edu/ (accessed May 24, 2012).

20. Houston Independent School District, "Michael E. DeBakey High School for Health Professions," http://schools.houstonisd.org/domain/10790 (accessed May 28, 2012).

21. University of Texas Medical Branch, "School of Nursing: 120 Years Young," *Impact Online*, March 16, 2010, http://www.utmb.edu/impact/?i=11 (accessed May 15, 2012).

22. Harris Health System, "About Us," https://www.hchdonline.com/en/about-us/pages/default.aspx (accessed May 28, 2012).

23. Texas Trauma Institute, Memorial Hermann, "The History of Life Flight," http://trauma.memorialhermann.org/life-flight/the-history-of-life-flight/ (accessed July 28, 2013).

24. Mizanur Rahman, "Memorial Hermann Hospital Starts New Trauma Institute," *Houston Chronicle*, May 29, 2012, http://blog.chron.com/newswatch/2012/05/memorial-hermann-hospital-starts-new-trauma-institute/ (accessed May 29, 2012). Memorial Hermann, "About Us," http://www.memorialhermann.org/aboutus/ (accessed May 29, 2012).

25. St. Luke's Episcopal Health System, "About Us: Our History," http://www.stlukestexas.com/AboutUs/OurHistory.cfm (accessed May 16, 2012).

26. Methodist Hospital System, "About Us," http://www.methodisthealth.com/body.cfm?id=36513 (accessed May 30, 2012); Methodist Hospital System, "Methodist DeBakey Heart & Vascular Center," http://www.methodisthealth.com/mdhvc.cfm?id=35826 (accessed May 30, 2012); Denton A. Cooley, *100,000 Hearts: A Surgeon's Memoir* (Austin: Dolph Briscoe Center for American History, University of Texas at Austin, 2012), 88–89, 146, 196–98.

27. Texas Children's Hospital, "History of Texas Children's Hospital," http://www.texaschildrens.org/About-Us/History/ (accessed June 6, 2012).

28. As a colonel during World War II, Dr. Michael DeBakey served on the Surgeon General's staff, earned the US Army Legion of Merit award, and conducted studies that led to the development of mobile army surgical hospitals, or MASH units. Pres. George W. Bush signed Public Law 108-170 on December 6, 2003, officially changing the name of the facility to the Michael E. DeBakey VA Medical Center. US Department of Veterans Affairs, "Michael E. DeBakey VA Medical Center–Houston,

Texas," http://www.houston.va.gov/about/aboutmedvamc_history.asp (accessed May 30, 2012).

29. Ronda Wendler, "Sabin Vaccine Institute Joins Texas Medical Center, Becomes 51st Member Institution," *Texas Medical Center News* 34, no. 10 (June 1, 2012), http://tmcnews.tendenci5production2.net/articles/sabin-vaccine-institute-joins-texas-medical-center-becomes-51st-member-institution/ (accessed July 30, 2012). Dr. Hotez is also a professor of pediatrics and molecular virology and microbiology and chief of the Pediatric Tropical Medicine section. In addition, he holds the Texas Children's Hospital Endowed Chair of Tropical Pediatrics. See Baylor College of Medicine, "Peter J. Hotez, M.D., Ph.D.," http://www.bcm.edu/tropicalmedicine/peter-hotez (accessed July 30, 2012).

30. "52nd Member Institution: DePelchin Children's Center Joins Texas Medical Center," *Texas Medical Center News* 34, no. 11 (June 15, 2012): 1; DePelchin Children's Center, "About Us," http://www.depelchin.org/About-DePelchin/About-De-Pelchin-211.html (accessed June 15, 2012).

31. Texas Medical Center, "The Texas Medical Center."

32. Richard E. Wainerdi, interview by William H. Kellar, June 7, 2010.

33. Richard E. Wainerdi, interview by William H. Kellar, May 10, 2012.

34. Ibid.

## Epilogue

1. Marguerite Johnston, *Houston: The Unknown City, 1836–1946* (College Station: Texas A&M University Press, 1991), 387. See also Joseph A. Pratt and Christopher J. Castaneda, *Builders: Herman and George R. Brown* (College Station: Texas A&M University Press, 1999), 278; Marvin Hurley, *Decisive Years for Houston* (Houston: Houston Chamber of Commerce, 1966), 415, 416, 420. City of Houston, "Houston Facts and Figures," http://www.houstontx.gov/abouthouston/houstonfacts.html (accessed April 12, 2012); Port of Houston Authority, "Overview," http://www.portofhouston.com/about-us/overview/ (accessed November 22, 2010).

2. By 1945, Anderson, Clayton & Company had 223 cotton gins, 33 cottonseed oil plants, and 123 warehouses worldwide. Thomas D. Anderson, "Anderson, Clayton and Company," *Handbook of Texas Online*, http://www.tshaonline.org/handbook/online/articles/dia01 (accessed November 22, 2010); John Fichter, interview by William H. Kellar, July 8, 2005.

3. W. Merrill Glasgow, interview by William H. Kellar, May 19, 2004, *This Is Anderson, Clayton & Co.* (Houston: Anderson, Clayton & Co, 1985), courtesy of Merrill Glasgow.

4. W. Merrill Glasgow, interview by William H. Kellar, May 19, 2004; "Quaker Gobbles Up Anderson Clayton," *Wall Street Journal*, October 1, 1986; *The Wall Street Journal*, December 2, 1987. Quaker Oats wanted the pet foods division and soon sold

all of the food division to Kraft Foods. This divesting continued the following year, when Quaker sold ACCO Feeds, Inc., to Cargill Incorporated and the Western Cotton Services Group to the Julien Group.

5. W. Merrill Glasgow, interview by William H. Kellar, May 19, 2004; Thomas D. Anderson, interview by William H. Kellar, December 11, 2003; Thomas D. Anderson, interview by William H. Kellar, February 9, 2006; John Fichter, interview by William H. Kellar, July 8, 2005; Gibson Gayle Jr., interview by Joseph A. Pratt, November 5, 2007.

6. M. D. Anderson Foundation, "Trust Indenture Creating the M. D. Anderson Foundation," 1936, 12, M. D. Anderson Foundation files.

7. Richard E. Wainerdi, interview by William H. Kellar, June 7, 2010; Gibson Gayle Jr., interview by William H. Kellar, February 17, 2010. The law firm has changed its names many times through the years. On June 1, 1940, it officially became Fulbright, Crooker, Freeman & Bates. See John H. Crooker Jr. and Gibson Gayle Jr., *Fulbright & Jaworski, 75 Years: 1919–1994* (Houston: Fulbright & Jaworski LLP, 1994), 51.

8. University of Houston, Board of Regents, "In Memoriam: Colonel William B. Bates," June 3, 1974, M. D. Anderson Foundation files; Newton Gresham (Philosophical Society of Texas), "William Bartholomew Bates, 1890–1974," M. D. Anderson Foundation files.

9. "Med Center Co-founder Dead at 93," *Houston Post,* July 14, 1980. Freeman echoed this sentiment to interviewer N. Don Macon, stating, "There can be a lot done if we are not too particular about who gets the credit for it." See N. Don Macon, *Mr. John H. Freeman and Friends: A Story of the Texas Medical Center and How It Began* (Houston: Texas Medical Center, 1973), 14.

10. Gibson Gayle Jr., interview by William H. Kellar, February 17, 2010; N. Don Macon, *South from Flower Mountain: A Conversation with William B. Bates* (Houston: Texas Medical Center, 1975), 59.

11. Gibson Gayle Jr., interview by Joseph A. Pratt, November 5, 2007; Richard E. Wainerdi, interview by William H. Kellar, June 7, 2010; Charles W. Hall, interview by William H. Kellar, February 15, 2010.

12. David M. Underwood, interview by William H. Kellar, April 20, 2012.

13. Gibson Gayle Jr., interview by William H. Kellar, February 17, 2010.

14. Adam Meyerson, "When Philanthropy Goes Wrong," *Wall Street Journal,* March 10, 2012; Martin Morse Wooster, "The Giving Game: The Saga of Philanthropy Still Needs Its History," *Weekly Standard,* May 14, 2012, 42–43. See also Olivier Zunz, *Philanthropy in America: A History* (Princeton: Princeton University Press, 2012); Jeffrey J. Cain, *Protecting Donor Intent: How to Define and Safeguard Your Philanthropic Principles* (N.p.: Philanthropy Roundtable, 2012); Richard E. Wainerdi, interview by William H. Kellar, June 7, 2010, and May 10, 2012.

# A Note on Sources

The secondary literature used in this study is cited in the endnotes that appear for each chapter. Primary research materials for this history came from several major sources, including the files of the M. D. Anderson Foundation, the McGovern Historical Collections and Research Center of the Houston Academy of Medicine–Texas Medical Center Library, the Houston Metropolitan Research Center of the Houston Public Library, and Special Collections, M. D. Anderson Library, University of Houston. In addition, W. Merrill Glasgow, former executive vice president of Anderson, Clayton & Company, graciously granted access to his collection of annual reports and other materials related to the firm.

There are several sources for the oral history interviews utilized in this project. First, these include interviews conducted between 2000 and 2012 by the author, William H. Kellar. In addition, the Texas Medical Center engaged historian Louis J. Marchiafava to conduct interviews with members of the board of trustees, and during 1973 N. Don Macon, University of Texas Health Science Center, Houston, conducted a series of videotaped interviews with many of the surviving founders and early participants in building the Texas Medical Center and its institutions. Additional interviews were conducted by William D. Seybold and by Joseph A. Pratt. Although some of the interviewees mentioned below are not directly quoted in the text, all provided important historical background information for this project.

## Interviews Conducted by William H. Kellar

| Name | Date of Interview |
|---|---|
| Thomas D. Anderson | January 26, 2000; December 11, 2003; February 9, 2006 |
| Billye Barlow | March 7, 2006 |
| Paul Gervais Bell | February 27, 2001; April 24, 2012 |
| Mary Bates Bentsen | August 23, 2010 |
| J. Searcy Bracewell Jr. | October 4, 2000 |
| Chester R. Burns, PhD | July 16, 2001 |
| William T. Butler, MD | September 9, 2010 |
| Denton A. Cooley, MD | December 26, 2000 |
| Michael E. DeBakey, MD | January 25, 2001 |
| John Fichter | July 8, 2005 |
| Gibson Gayle Jr. | February 17, 2010 |
| W. Merrill Glasgow | May 19, 2004 |
| Fenton Guinee | July 11, 2005 |
| Charles W. Hall | February 15, 2010 |
| Mavis P. Kelsey Sr., MD | September 19, 2000; February 7, 2001; December 11, 2003 |
| Avery "Buck" Newland | September 5, 2005 |
| William D. Seybold, MD | November 14, 2000 |
| David M. Underwood | April 20, 2012 |
| Richard E. Wainerdi, PhD | November 16, 2000; June 7, 2010; May 10, 2012 |
| C. W. Wellen | December 10, 2005 |

## Interviews Conducted by N. Don Macon

| Name | Date of Interview |
| --- | --- |
| W. Leland Anderson | October 9, 1973 |
| Hines H. Baker | September 21, 1973 |
| William B. Bates | April 19, 1973 |
| Julia Bertner Naylor | October 4, 1973 |
| R. Lee Clark, MD | November 30, 1973 |
| Frederick C. Elliott, DDS | July 19, 1973 |
| Ella Fondren | October 25, 1973 |
| John H. Freeman | August 2, 1973 |
| Earl C. Hankamer | October 9, 1973 |
| William A. Kirkland | September 20, 1973 |

## Interviews Conducted by Louis J. Marchiafava

| Name | Date of Interview |
| --- | --- |
| Thomas D. Anderson | May 4, 2000 |
| Daniel C. Arnold | August 1, 2001 |
| Paul Gervais Bell Jr. | June 28, 2001 |
| Jack S. Blanton | February 27, 2001 |
| Searcy Bracewell | September 10, 2001 |
| Holcombe Crosswell | June 26, 2000 |
| Gibson Gayle Jr. | March 23, 2001 |
| Charles W. Hall | May 23, 2005 |
| Philip Hoffman, PhD | October 3, 2000 |
| Richard J. V. Johnson | February 2, 2001 |
| John Kelsey, MD | August 27, 2001 |
| Mavis P. Kelsey Sr., MD | July 31, 2001 |
| Ben F. Love | March 21, 2001 |
| David M. Underwood | October 2, 2002 |

## Interviews Conducted by Joseph A. Pratt

| Name | Date of Interview |
|------|-------------------|
| Gibson Gayle | November 5, 2007 |

## Interviews Conducted by William D. Seybold

| Name | Date of Interview |
|------|-------------------|
| Frederick C. Elliott, DDS | August 9, 1971 |
| John H. Freeman | April 8, 1971 |
| Anna Hanselman | May 16, 1970 |

# Index

African Americans, 18, 55–56, 94, 141, 146–47, 157

Allen, Augustus C., 1, 2

Allen, John Kirby, 1, 2

American Cancer Society, 129

American Cotton Company, 29, 30–31, 32–33, 36

Amerman, A. Earl, 56

Anderson, Burdine (née Clayton), 26, 27, 28–29, 45–46, 75

Anderson, Clayton & Company: alliance with Fulbright, Crooker, Freeman & Bates, 47, 48, 61–62, 63–65; buyout clause, 67–68; direct connections in foreign markets, 36–37; establishment of, xxiii, 27–34; at foundation establishment, 66; founders' backgrounds, 24–27; Fulbright's initial connection to, 49–50; growth of, 37, 43–47; Houston location's advantages for, 37, 44, 49–50; influence in cotton industry, 64; initial advantages of, 34–36; as joint stock association, 45, 67–68; leadership's effectiveness, 41; move to Houston, 37–38; post-WWII fate of, 189–90; stock donation for Texas Children's Hospital, 156; and transportation improvements, 43; warehousing expansion, 44–45; work ethic of, 41–42

Anderson, Frank Ervin, 24–30, 34, 43, 45–46

Anderson, Hugh, 29

Anderson, James (Monroe's nephew), 69, 72

Anderson, James (no relation), 123, 142

Anderson, James Wisdom, 25

Anderson, Mary Ellen (née Dunaway), 25

Anderson, Monroe Dunaway: Bates's recollections of, 64–65, 81–82; Bender Hotel, move to, 42–43; character of, 29, 38, 40–41, 69, 72–73; contributions to company, 34, 36; daily activities near end of life, 70–71; death of, 73–74; estate planning, 65, 66–67; filing of will, 74–75; and foundation establishment, xxi, 66; friendships, 40–41; and Fulbright, 50–51; health problems, 68, 70, 71–72, 215n 10; Houston's opportunities for, xxiii; legacy of, 23, 185, 190–91, 192, 198–99; loyalty to company employees, 68; management style, 41; move into cotton industry, 27–28, 29–30; move to Houston, 38; origins of, 25, 27–28, 29; photos, 42, 71; public credit for medical center, 120; public health interest of, 68–69; social life of, 46; work ethic of, 41–42

Anderson, Neil, 26–27, 29

Anderson, Phillip, 4

Anderson, Thomas D.: on Anderson, Clayton's Oklahoma City location, 45; as executor, 69; on Frank's distaste for Galveston, 43; on Frank's family origins, 26; on Frank's talent for grading cotton, 36; on investment suggestions for Monroe's fortune, 74–75; and Monroe's health problems, 70, 71–73

Anderson, W. Leland, 69, 72, 123, *124*, 145, 162

Anderson-Clayton Securities Corporation, 67–68

Andrews, Ball, and Streetman, 49

Anti-Rat Society, 4

Arabia Temple Shrine Crippled Children's Clinic, 140–41

Bailey, Joseph Weldon, 63

Baker, James A., 84

Baker, Newton D., 54

Baker Memorial Pavilion, 79–80

banking industry: Anderson, Clayton's need for solid, 37–38; Andersons' origins in, 25, 29; in early 1900s Houston, 37–38; Monroe's investments, 40; State National Bank of Houston, 52, 63, 75, 213*n*5

Baptist Church, 99, 100, 101–2, 111, 154

Baptist Sanitarium (later Hospital), 16–17

Bates, James Madison, 57

Bates, Mary Frances (née Cook), 57

Bates, William Bartholomew: on Baylor medical school move, 104, 109, 116; on Bertner's predictions for value of medical center, 122; on cancer hospital development, 80, 84; death and legacy of, 192–94; foundation

establishment role of, 68–69; friendship with Monroe, 40; on history of medical center, 151; and Jaworski, 154; joining of law firm, 62–63; on loans to African American churches, 147; medical center development role, 115, 125, *193*; on meeting Anderson, Clayton partners, 64; on Monroe, 81–82; partnership status at law firm, 75; profile of, 56–63, *59*; recollections of Monroe, 64–65, 81–82; talent and experience of, 64; on Wilkins, 146

Bay City, 58

Baylor (University) College of Medicine: and city-county hospital debate, 157; current functions of, 170–71; and medical center, 103–10, 153–55; mid-20th century construction, 153–55; move to Houston, xxiv, 103–13, 116; origins of, 98–99; separation from Baylor University, 170; Southwestern Medical Foundation merger, 99–103

Baylor Dental College, 108

Baylor International Pediatric AIDS Initiative (BIPAI), 179

Baylor University trustees, 104–8, 112

Bellows, Warren S., 127, 147–48

Bender, E. L., 42–43

Bender, Frank V., 42–43

Bender Hotel, 42–43

Ben Taub General Hospital, 143, 157–58, *158*, 176

Bering brothers, 7

Bertner, Anna (née Miller), 86

Bertner, Ernst W.: address on medical center, 121–22, 222*n*9; Baylor medical school move to Houston, xxiv, 109; and cancer hospital development, 83, 86, 91–94, 117–20, 126; cancer illness of, 131–34; character of, 87–88; death and legacy of, 134–36; on foundation's relationship to institutions, 111; on library's importance to medical center, 140; at medical center dedication, 123; medical center development role, 117; photos, *91, 124, 134*; as president and promoter of medical center, xxiv–xxv, 126, 128–29, 130–31, 132–33; profile of, 86–91; and search for medical center location, 113–15

Bertner, Gus, 86–88

Bertner, Julia (née Williams), 90, 91, *92*

BIPAI (Baylor International Pediatric AIDS Initiative), 179

blacks, 18, 55–56, 94, 141, 146–47, 157

boards of trustees. *See* trustees

Boyles, T. J., 15

Brays Bayou Flood Control Project, 166–67

Bremond, Paul, 5, 6, 11

Briscoe, S. M., 20

Buffalo Bayou, 11, 20

Butler, P. P., *134*

Butler, William T., 109, 116

Callender, David L., 175

Campbell, Meyer, and Freeman, 52

Campbell, Thomas M., 87

Camp Logan, 54–55, 56

Camp Strake, 152

cancer, 76–78, 90, 131–34. *See also* M. D. Anderson Hospital for Cancer Research

Carter, William S., 88

Cary, Edward H., 99–102

Cash, William, 58

Cato, Arthur, 76, 118, 148

Center for Advanced Biomedical Imaging Research, 170

charitable foundation. *See* M. D. Anderson Foundation

charity health care: Ben Taub General Hospital, 143, 157–58, *158*, 176; caring for cancer patients, 78; Crippled Children's Clinic, 141; Jefferson Davis Hospital, 18, 84, 158, 176, 209n 30; medical center contribution to, 183; Speech and Hearing Center, 140; St. Joseph's Infirmary, 15, 156, 209n 25. *See also* Hermann Hospital

city-county hospitals: Ben Taub General Hospital, 143, 157–58, *158*, 176; Jefferson Davis Hospital, 18, 84, 158, 176, 209n 30

City of Houston Department of Health and Human Services, 180

civic virtue in Houston, xxii, 1, 24, 187–88. *See also* philanthropy

civil rights movement, 156–57

Civil War, 11, 14, 25

Clark, R. Lee, 126–27, 132, *193*

Clayton, Benjamin: Bates's recollections of, 64; contribution to company, 33–35, 36–37; departure from Anderson, Clayton, 67; and establishment of company, 32; origins of, 31; shipping improvements, 43

Clayton, Dessie Burdine (Mrs. F. E. Anderson), 26, 27, 28–29, 45–46, 75

Clayton, Fletcher (née Burdine), 30

Clayton, James Monroe, 30

Clayton, Julia, 43

Clayton, Sue (née Vaughan), 156

Clayton, William Lockhart: Bates's recollections of, 64; and buyout problem
upon Monroe's death, 68; contribution to company, 34–35; and establishment of company, 29–30, 32–33;
and Fleming, 40, 212*n* 30; market
knowledge of, 36; on Monroe's death,
73; move to Houston, 43; profile of,
30, *32*
Cody, Claude C. Jr., 18, 111
Collins, Carr P., 102, 104–6
Columbia HCA Healthcare Corporation,
164–65
Committee on Cancer, 78
Cooley, Denton A., 178
cotton industry, 6, 8–13, 20–21,
25–29, 35, 44–45. *See also* Anderson, Clayton & Company
Crooker, John H.: Camp Logan court-
martial, 56; founding of law firm,
48, 61; judge advocate experience,
63; political career, 53–54; profile of,
52–56, *57*; prostitution close-down
case, 54–55; talent and experience
of, 63
Crooker, Margaret (née Kelton), 53
Crooker, Norman W., 53
Cullen, Hugh Roy and Lillie, 129, 149
Cullen, Thomas, 90
Cullen Building, 129–30, *130*
Cullinan, Joseph S., 18, 153

Dallas, and Baylor University College of
Medicine, 106
DeBakey, Michael, 178, 229–30*n* 28
deed restrictions in medical center, challenge to, 164–65
Dental Branch at Houston, UT. *See* University of Texas School of Dentistry
dental schools, 81, 93, 95–96, 108,

141, 143–44. *See also* University of
Texas School of Dentistry
DePelchin Children's Center, 182
desegregation in Houston, 157
de Zavala, Lorenzo, 3
doctors. *See* physician community
drugstores, 6
Dudley, Ray L., 112, 123
Duke, James "Red," 153
Dunaway, Mary Ellen (Mrs. J. W. Ander-
son), 25
Duncan Neurological Research Insti-
tute, 179
Dunn Helistop, 153

Eastwood, Richard T., 159, 160, 162
Eldridge, John W., 4
Elkins, James A., 56
Elliott, Frederick C.: affiliation of dental
school into UT system, 95–96; on
Bertner's address on medical center,
121–22, 222*n* 9; character of, 143;
and city-county hospital debate,
157; in director position at medical
center, xxv, 137, 141–43, 145; and
governance of medical center, 109;
medical center development role, 79,
93, 117, 156; photo, *193*; profile
of, 143–45; public health role in
Houston, 22; on Rainey's challenge
to medical center, 120; retirement
of, 158–59; on Spies's desire to move
medical school, 83
Ennis, Cornelius, 5, 6, 11
European role in cotton market, 35, 36,
44
Ewing, Alexander, 4
Ewing, T. J. Jr., 56
experimental treatment, as hallmark of
cancer center, 133–34

federal matching funds for medical
    center projects, 154–55
Fichter, John, 190
Fisher, Arthur, 40, 70–71
Fisher House, 180
Fleming, Clare, 40
Fleming, Lamar Jr., 40, 68, 152, 212*n*
    30, 219*n* 14
Fleming, Lamar Sr., 32
flooding threat to medical center, 166,
    167–68, 172–73, 228*n* 9
Foster, John, 18
Freeman, James D., 51
Freeman, John Henry: and Baylor
    medical school move, 103–4; on
    Bertner's contribution, 93, 135; on
    cancer hospital development, 79–80;
    charter for medical center, 122; on
    crippled children's clinic, 141; death
    and legacy of, 194; foundation estab-
    lishment role, 68–69; and Fulbright,
    49; and governance of medical
    center, 109; joining of law firm, 63;
    medical center development role, 93,
    115, 125–26; and Monroe, 40; nam-
    ing of building for, 171, 173; photos,
    52, 195; profile of, 51–52, 63; talent
    and experience, 63
Freeman, Rose (née Phelps), 51
Fulbright, Bertie (née Welborn), 48–49
Fulbright, Clarence, xxiii
Fulbright, Crooker, Freeman & Bates: al-
    liance with Anderson, Clayton, 47, 48,
    61–62, 63–65; development of firm,
    48, 61; estate planning for Monroe,
    66–67; foundation role of, 48; Jawor-
    ski's joining of, 154; legacy of, 191–92.
    See also *principal partners by name*
Fulbright, Rufus Clarence, 48, 49–51,
    50, 61, 103

Fulbright, Rufus T., 48–49
Fulbright & Jaworski LLP. *See* Fulbright,
    Crooker, Freeman & Bates
fund-raising for Texas Medical Center,
    125, 154–55, 156

Galveston: Andersons' exploratory trip,
    43; and debate on cancer hospital
    location, 80–81; economic competi-
    tion with Houston, 10, 11, 12, 13,
    21; hurricanes, 21, 168
Garcia, Carolyn Clause, 165
Garrow, H. W., 12
Gayle, Gibson, 192, 194, 196
George Hermann Estate case, 56
Glasgow, Merrill, 189
Goar, Everett L., 18, 110
governance. *See* trustees
Grant, Ulysses S., 77
Graves, Joe Henry, 72
Graves, Marvin L., 18, 112
Great Depression, 62, 66, 67–68, 99
Greenwood, James, 18, 72
Gresham, Newton, 193–94
Gribble, R. D., 12
Gulf Coast Regional Blood Center, 180

Hall, Charles W., 192, 196
Hankamer, Earl C., 113
Hanselman, Anna, 117–18, 119
Harris County Hospital District (HCHD),
    176, 226–27*n* 29
Harris County Medical Society (HCMS),
    14, 110–12
Harris County Psychiatric Center, 172
Harris Health System, 176
Hart, James P., 138–39
Harvin, William C., 162
HCHD (Harris County Hospital District),
    176, 226–27*n* 29

HCMS (Harris County Medical Society), 14, 110–12

health care: Houston's early history, 2–4, 13–17; philanthropic role in, 24, 68–69. *See also* M. D. Anderson Foundation; public health

Health Science Center, UT, 127, 171–72

Hedgecroft Clinic and Hospital, 18–19

Heights Clinic Hospital, 209*n* 29

heliport, 153, 176–77

Hermann, George, 56

Hermann Hospital: challenge to medical center's nonprofit status, 165; establishment of, 18, *19*; flooding of, 167; heliport, 153, 176–77; and Hermann estate complications, 56; and land for medical school, 114; leasing of beds to cancer hospital, 94; post-WWII expansion, 129, 130

Hermann Professional Building, 129, 130

High School for Health Professions (HSHP), 174–75

Hill, George A. Jr., 124, 125

Hill, Jerome, 30

HISD (Houston Independent School District), 174–75

*A History of Baylor University College of Medicine* (Moursund), 100

Hoffman, Philip G., 162, 193

Hogg, Mike, 80

Hogg, Will, 80

Holcomb, John B., 177

Holcombe, Oscar, 18

Hospital Laundry Cooperative Association, 163

hospitals, 14–19, 79, 111. See also *individual hospitals by name*

Hotez, Peter, 181, 230*n* 29

House, Thomas William, 5, 6–7

Houston: advantages for Anderson, Clayton, 37, 44, 49–50; Allen brothers' promotion of, 2; Anderson, Clayton's move to, 37–38; attractions for Bertner, 89; Baylor medical school's move to, xxiv, 103–13, 116; Benjamin Clayton in, 31; as cancer hospital site, 80–82; civic virtue in, xxii, 1, 24, 187–88; civil rights movement, 156–57; cotton industry, 8–13; cultural venue growth, 44; early medical care developments, 2–3, 4–5, 13–20, 22, 209*n* 29; economic growth, xxi, 10, 37–38, 188; entrepreneurial spirit in, xxi–xxii, 1, 5–7, 24; founding of, 1–2; vs. Galveston, 10, 11, 12, 13, 21; oil industry's impact on, 37; population growth in, 7, 9, 13, 20; pre-Civil War/Republic era, 2–11; red-light district, 54–55; sanitation improvements, 4, 19–22

Houston, Sam, 2

Houston Academy of Medicine–Texas Medical Center Library, 140, 181

Houston and Texas Central Railroad, 6

Houston Cotton Exchange, 6, 12–13, 20, 37, *39*, 45

Houston Endowment, 154

Houston Eye, Ear, Nose, and Throat Hospital, 18

Houston Heights, 209*n* 29

Houston Independent School District (HISD), 174–75

Houston Infirmary, 14–15

Houston Junior League, 70

Houston Negro Hospital (later Riverside Hospital), 18

Houston Negro Hospital Nursing School, 18

Houston Ship Channel, 10–13, 20–21
Houston State Psychiatric Institute for Research and Training, 152–53
Howard, A. Philo, 16
HSHP (High School for Health Professions), 174–75
Humphries, David, 54
hurricanes, 58, 167–68
Hutchins, William J., 5

infectious diseases, 4, 5, 19–20
inheritances, 46, 74–75
Institute of Religion, 150
insurance law, 87

Jachimczyk Forensic Center, 181
Jan and Dan Duncan Neurological Research Institute, 179
Jaworski, Leon, 153–54, *155*, 162, 226*n* 24
Jefferson Davis Hospital, 18, 84, 158, 176, 209*n* 30
Jesse H. Jones Clinical Research Building, 154
Jesse H. Jones Rotary House International, 169–70
Jewish Institute for Medical Research, 154
Jim Crow segregation laws, 55–56
John P. McGovern Commons, 166
John P. McGovern Museum of Health and Medical Science, 181
John S. Dunn Helistop, 153
Johnson, Richard J. V., 162
joint stock association, 45, 67–68
Jones, Anson, 3
Jones, Jesse H., 38, 89, 133, *134*, 140, 154
Joseph A. Jachimczyk Forensic Center, 181

Kelsey, Mavis P., 132
Kendall, Clarence, 54
Keyes, E. L., 88, 89
Kidd, George W., 12
Kimball, George W., 6
Kipp, H. A., 119
Knox, R. W., 17
Kokernot, H. L., 102–3, 105–6
Kyle, J. Allen, 16

Larendon, George W., 20
Larendon, Joshua, 14–15
Latin America, medical center as resource for, 128–29
laundry facility, 164
Law, Francis Marion, 118
lawyers/legal team and trustee role. *See* Fulbright, Crooker, Freeman & Bates
Levy, Moise D., 112
libraries, 140, 152, 181
Life Flight service, 153, 176–77
LifeGift Organ Donation Center, 181
Logue, Lyle J., 18
Lyndon B. Johnson General Hospital (LBJ), 176

*Making Cancer History* (Olson), 133
Malone, Clarence, 40, 70
managed care, threat to nonprofit status, 164–65
Martin, D. K., 102–3, 104–6
Martin, James A., 38
Martin, James M., 78
Massey, Otis, 22
Mays, L. T., 16
McGovern Commons, 166
McGovern Museum of Health and Medical Science, 181
M. D. Anderson Foundation: accolades for, 120, 150; Anderson Basic

M. D. Anderson Foundation (*cont.*)
Research Building funding, 154;
Baylor medical school move, 103–9,
111–12, 116; cancer hospital
establishment, 22–23, 66, 78–82,
83–85, 91–94, 97, 125, 145, 151;
cancer hospital support, 127; dental
school funding, 96, 141; distinguish-
ing from cancer hospital, xxvi–xxvii;
establishment of, xxiii, 65, 68–69;
Fulbright law partners' role in
establishing, 65; healthcare support
beyond medical center, 125–26;
historical overview (1956), 151–52;
initial contributions, 70; Institute of
Religion funding, 150; legacy of, 74,
160, 182, 187–99; library funding, 140; loans to African American
churches, 146–47; management
and administration of, 146–47, 156;
medical center development role, 83,
113–16, 122–25, 139; Monroe's
role in, 70; purposes of, 69; resources
of, 195–96; Speech and Hearing
Center funding, 153; transfer of
wealth upon Monroe's death, 74–75;
trustees and governance, 69, 70, 75,
145–48, 197–98

M. D. Anderson Hospital for Cancer Research (later Cancer Center): current
functions of, 169–70; distinguish-
ing from M. D. Anderson Foundation, xxvi–xxvii; establishment of,
91–94, 97; expansions of, 127, *128*,
137–41, *138*, 148–49, 150–51,
156, 169; foundation's role in
creating, 22–23, 66, 78–82, 83–85,
91–94, 97, 125, 145, 151; middle-
class focus of, 78–79; at The Oaks,
84–85, *85*, 94, 117, 119; planning

for location of, 80–81, 83–86, 93;
post-WWII development, 131;
preparations for operation, 117–18;
search for first permanent director,
126–27

M. D. Anderson Memorial Library, 152
Medical and Surgical Society of Hous-
ton, 4
medical care. *See* health care
medical ethics, 150
medical training programs: High School
for Health Professions, 174–75;
initial 19th-century, 15–16; mental
health, 152–53; nursing schools, 16,
18, 173–74; UT Medical School at
Houston, 167, 171–73, *172*, 176.
*See also* Baylor (University) College of
Medicine; dental schools
*Medicine in Greater Houston: 1836–1956*
(Moursund), 4
MEDVAMC (Veterans Affairs Medical
Center), 179–80
Memorial Healthcare System, 165
Memorial Hermann Healthcare System
(later Memorial Hermann-TMC), 16,
177
Memorial Hospital in New York, 77
Memorial Hospital School of Nursing,
16
Menninger Clinic, 170–71
mental health facilities, 152–53, 171,
172
mercantile businesses in pre-Civil War
Houston, 6–7
Methodist Hospital, 17, 140, 150–51,
156, 178
Michael E. DeBakey Veterans Affairs
Medical Center (MEDVAMC), 179–80
Moody, Daniel J., 61
Moody, George H., 18

Moore, Francis Jr., 4

Morrow, Wright, 149

Moursund, Walter H.: and Baylor medical school move, 99, 100–102, 106, 110–13; on early hospitals in Houston, 15; on early Houston's public health issues, 4; photos, *101, 134*

museum, 181

Musgrove, John, 94

Nabisco building, renovation and reuse of, 166

National Center for Human Performance (NCHP), 168

Neff, Pat, 104, 105–6

New England's role in cotton market, 35

New York Cancer Hospital, 77

New York's role in cotton market, 35

Norsworthy, Oscar L., 16

Norton Rose Fulbright, 192

not-for-profit principle, challenge to, 164–65

nursing training programs, 16, 18, 173–74

The Oaks, 84–85, *85*, 94, 117, 119

Ochsner, Alton, 127, 132, 135

oil industry, 37

Oklahoma City, 27, 35, 37, 43

Oldham, Dudley Y., 131

Olson, James S., 84, 133

Olson, John V., 143

OrNda Healthcorp, 165

Page, David, 165

Painter, Theophilus S., 125, 126–27

Parkland Hospital, Dallas, 106

Park View Hospital, 18

Peveto, D. R., 16

pharmacology, 87, 174

philanthropy: and foundation's legacy, 74, 197–98; in health care development, 24, 68–69; Houston's tradition of, 187–88; Monroe's quite style of, 41, 70. *See also* M. D. Anderson Foundation

physician community, 4, 13–14, 16, 78, 110–12

Physician's and Surgeon's Hospital Company of Houston, 16

politics, 53–54, 61, 62, 121

Polk, Sam, 62

population growth in Houston, 7, *9*, 13, 20

Port of Houston, 37, 43, 44–45

Prairie View A&M University College of Nursing, 174

Pressler, Herman P., 162

prostitution case, Crooker's, 54–55

psychiatric health facilities, 152–53, 171, 172

public health: early focus due to Houston's location, 2–3, 4–5; Elliott's dedication to causes of, 144; first half of 20th century, 19–23; infectious disease threat, 4, 5, 19–20; Monroe's long-term interest in, 68–69. *See also* charity health care

Public Health Institute of Houston, 22

Quentin R. Mease Community Hospital, 176

Quin, Clinton S., 118, 149

racial segregation, 18, 94, 141, 146–47, 157

racism, Camp Logan's black soldier's revolt, 55–56

railroad industry: Benjamin Clayton's knowledge of, 31; Fulbright's

railroad industry (*cont.*)
  background with, 49, 50–51;
  railroad hospitals, 14–15, 17; role in
  Houston's development, 6, 9–10, 13
Rainey, Homer, 80, 86, 105, 111,
  119–21
Ralston, W. W., 16, 18
red-light district, Houston, 54–55
Republic of Texas, 2–7
rhabdomyosarcoma, 131–32
Rice, Horace Baldwin, 12
Rice, William Marsh, 5, 6, 11, 84
Rice Hotel, 89, 90
Rice Institute (later University), 84,
  152, 174
Robbins, Robert C., 185
Roberts, T. E., 73–74
Robertson Pavilion, 130
Ronald McDonald House, 179, 180
Rudisill, Ida J., 16
Rudisill Sanitarium (later Memorial
  Hospital), 16

Sabin Vaccine Institute, 181
Sampson, J. H., 16
sanitation in Houston, 4, 19–22
San Jacinto, 3
Santa Anna, Antonio Lopez de, 3
Scott, J. W., 20
Sealy, Tom, 148
Settegast, J. J., 56
Seybold, William D., 135
Shearn, Charles, 6
ship channel development, 10–13,
  20–21
Sisters of Charity of the Incarnate
  Word, 15, 209n 25
Slataper, Felician J., 20
Sloan-Kettering Institute, 77
Smith, Ashbel, 4

Smyth, Cheves M., 171
Southern Pacific Hospital (later Hospital
  Assoc. of SP Lines in TX and LA),
  17–18
Southwestern Medical Foundation,
  99–103, 106
Speech and Hearing Center, 140, 153
Spies, John, 78, 80, 81, 85–86,
  217–18n 2
State National Bank of Houston, 52, 63,
  75, 213n 5
Sterrett, John H., 11
Stevens, W. A., 16
Stevenson, Coke, 118
Steward, John S., 56
Stewart, George D., 88–89
St. Joseph's Infirmary (later Hospital),
  15–16, 156, 209n 25
St. Luke's Episcopal Hospital, 139, 140,
  149, 156, 164–65, 178–79, 225n
  17
Strauss, William, 22
Stuart, David F., 14–15
Sutherland, John, 3

Taub, Ben, 157–58
tax laws and creation of foundation,
  68, 75
Taylor, Judson, 86, 110
TECO (Thermal Energy Corporation),
  163
Texas A&M University, 174
Texas Children's Hospital, 129, 139,
  145, 156, 178, 179
Texas Dental College, 81, 93, 143–44
Texas Exes, 125
Texas Heart Institute, 178–79
Texas Medical Association, 78
Texas Medical Center: Baylor medical
  school as component of, 103–10,

153–55; cancer hospital as catalyst for, 93; challenges to collaborative community model, 164–65, 227n 5; charter for, 122–23; city-county hospital debate, 157; current reach and reputation, 161–85; dedicatory dinner, 123–25; defining function of, xxv–xxvi; dental college's role in, 95–96; Eastwood appointment, 159; economic impact of, 183; Elliott's dream for, 79; equal admissions policy, 157; flooding threat to, 166, 167–68, 172–73, 228n 9; Freeman's role in, 93, 109, 115, 122, 125–26; fund-raising for, 125, 154–55, 156; heating and cooling plant, 164; Hurricane Katrina assistance, 167; independence of, 109; initial conceptions, 22–23, 83; initial string of events leading to, 75–76; land acquisition pattern, 162; and Latin America, 128–29; laundry facility, 164; McGovern Commons and Campus, 166; mid-20th-century expansion of, 137–41, 146, *147*, 148–56; naming of, 109; permanent location for, 113–16; photo, *184*; post-WWII development, 125–26, 129–31, 132–33; pulling together of components (1940s), 103–4; research initiatives, 168; rise in national prominence of, 150; 21st-century development, 165–66, 183–85; UT's centralization challenge to, 119–21. *See also* Bertner, Ernst W.; Elliott, Frederick C.; M. D. Anderson Foundation

Texas Medical Center, Inc. (TMC): charter for, 122–23; current function of, 161–69, 183–84; relationship to Texas Medical Center, xxv–xxvi; trustees and governance, 123, 136, 145, 159, 162. *See also* Bertner, Ernst W.; Elliott, Frederick C.

Texas Medical Center South Campus, 170

Texas Southern University (TSU), 174

Texas State Board of Medical Examiners, 14

Texas State Hotel, 70, 72

Texas Trauma Institute, 177

Texas Women's University (TWU), 173–74

The (formerly Texas) Institute for Rehabilitation and Research (TIRR Memorial Hermann), 152, 177–78

Thermal Energy Corporation (TECO), 163

TMC (Texas Medical Center, Inc.). *See* Texas Medical Center, Inc. (TMC)

transportation, 6, 7–8, 10–13, 20–21, 43. *See also* railroad industry

Tropical Storm Allison, 167, 172–73

trustees: Baylor University, 104–8, 112; M. D. Anderson Foundation, 69, 70, 75, 145–48, 197–98; Texas Medical Center, Inc., 123, 136, 145, 159, 162

TWU (Texas Women's University), 173–74

UH College of Pharmacy, 174

Underwood, David M., xxvi, 162, 196–97

United States, Texas' annexation by, 3

University Cancer Foundation, UT, 151

University of Houston (UH), 152, 174

University of Texas (UT): and Baylor medical school move to Houston, 105; and cancer hospital plans, 78,

University of Texas (UT) (*cont.*)
80–81, 83–84, 86, 93; dental school
affiliation, 95–96; foundation's
matching funding scheme for medi-
cal center, 125; proposal to move all
units to Austin, 119–21
University of Texas Health Science
Center at Houston (UTHealth), 127,
171–72
University of Texas M. D. Anderson
Cancer Center. *See* M. D. Anderson
Hospital for Cancer Research
University of Texas Medical Branch at
Galveston (UTMB), 80–81, 86, 175
University of Texas Medical School at
Houston, 167, 171–73, *172*, 176
University of Texas School of Dentistry,
139, 141, 142, 144, 150, 157, 173
UT. *See* University of Texas (UT)
UTHealth (University of Texas Health
Science Center at Houston), 127,
171–72
UTMB (University of Texas Medical
Branch at Galveston), 80–81, 86,
175

vaccine institute, 181
Veterans Affairs Medical Center (MED-
VAMC), 179–80
Veteran's Hospital, 139–40
Vinson & Elkins, 62

Wainerdi, Richard E.: on decentraliza-
tion of facilities, 183; on DePelchin
Children's Center, 182; on medical

center's legacy, 198; on medical
center's reputation, 185; as president
of TMC, 162, *163*, 168, 175
water transportation, 10–13, 20–21
Welch, Robert A., 70
White, A. R., *134*
Wilkins, Eunice (née Lewis), 75
Wilkins, Horace M.: and Baylor medical
school move to Houston, 109; and
cancer hospital development, 80; as
foundation trustee, 70, 75; illness
and death of, 145–46; and medical
center location, 115; other positions
held, 216n 18; profile of, 75, *76*; and
State National Bank, 52
Wilkins, John A., 52
Wilkins, W. G., 75
will, filing of Monroe's, 74–75
Williams, Jack Kenney, 162
Williams, Julia (Mrs. E. W. Bertner), 90,
91, *92*
Woodward, Dudley Jr., 120, 126
World War I, 21, 44–45, 54–55, 56,
58–60, 89
World War II: construction restrictions
during, 82, 83, 94, 116, 118; ending
of, 122; physician shortage during,
100, 113
Wortham, Gus, 153
Wright Clinic and Hospital, 18

yellow fever, 5
York, J. B., 20
Young, Hugh H., 89, 90